Surgical Advances in Ankle Arthritis

Editor

ALAN NG

CLINICS IN PODIATRIC MEDICINE AND SURGERY

www.podiatric.theclinics.com

Consulting Editor
THOMAS ZGONIS

October 2017 • Volume 34 • Number 4

ELSEVIER

1600 John F. Kennedy Boulevard • Suite 1800 • Philadelphia, Pennsylvania, 19103-2899

http://www.theclinics.com

CLINICS IN PODIATRIC MEDICINE AND SURGERY Volume 34, Number 4
October 2017 ISSN 0891-8422, ISBN-13: 978-0-323-54686-7

Editor: Lauren Boyle
Developmental Editor: Meredith Madeira

Photocopying
Single photocopies of single articles may be made for personal use as allowed by national copyright laws. Permission of the Publisher and payment of a fee is required for all other photocopying, including multiple or systematic copying, copying for advertising or promotional purposes, resale, and all forms of document delivery. Special rates are available for educational institutions that wish to make photocopies for non-profit educational classroom use. For information on how to seek permission visit www.elsevier.com/permissions or call: (+44) 1865 843830 (UK)/(+1) 215 239 3804 (USA).

Derivative Works
Subscribers may reproduce tables of contents or prepare lists of articles including abstracts for internal circulation within their institutions. Permission of the Publisher is required for resale or distribution outside the institution. Permission of the Publisher is required for all other derivative works, including compilations and translations (please consult www.elsevier.com/permissions).

Electronic Storage or Usage
Permission of the Publisher is required to store or use electronically any material contained in this periodical, including any article or part of an article (please consult www.elsevier.com/permissions). Except as outlined above, no part of this publication may be reproduced, stored in a retrieval system or transmitted in any form or by any means, electronic, mechanical, photocopying, recording or otherwise, without prior written permission of the Publisher.

Notice
No responsibility is assumed by the Publisher for any injury and/or damage to persons or property as a matter of products liability, negligence or otherwise, or from any use or operation of any methods, products, instructions or ideas contained in the material herein. Because of rapid advances in the medical sciences, in particular, independent verification of diagnoses and drug dosages should be made.

Although all advertising material is expected to conform to ethical (medical) standards, inclusion in this publication does not constitute a guarantee or endorsement of the quality or value of such product or of the claims made of it by its manufacturer.

Clinics in Podiatric Medicine and Surgery (ISSN 0891-8422) is published quarterly by Elsevier Inc., 360 Park Avenue South, New York, NY 10010-1710. Months of issue are January, April, July, and October. Business and Editorial Offices: 1600 John F. Kennedy Blvd., Ste. 1800, Philadelphia, PA 19103-2899. Customer Service Office: 3251 Riverport Lane, Maryland Heights, MO 63043. Periodicals postage paid at New York, NY and additional mailing offices. Subscription prices are $288.00 per year for US individuals, $518.00 per year for US institutions, $100.00 per year for US students and residents, $374.00 per year for Canadian individuals, $626.00 for Canadian institutions, $439.00 for international individuals, $626.00 per year for international institutions and $220.00 per year for Canadian and foreign students/residents. To receive student/resident rate, orders must be accompanied by name of affiliated institution, date of term, and the *signature* of program/residency coordinator on institution letterhead. Orders will be billed at individual rate until proof of status is received. Foreign air speed delivery is included in all *Clinics* subscription prices. All prices are subject to change without notice. POSTMASTER: Send address changes to *Clinics in Podiatric Medicine and Surgery*, Elsevier Health Sciences Division, Subscription Customer Service, 3251 Riverport Lane, Maryland Heights, MO 63043. **Customer Service: 1-800-654-2452 (US). From outside of the US, call 314-447-8871. Fax: 314-447-8029. E-mail: JournalsCustomerService-usa@elsevier.com (for print support); JournalsOnlineSupport-usa@elsevier. com (for online support).**

Reprints. For copies of 100 or more of articles in this publication, please contact the Commercial Reprints Department, Elsevier Inc., 360 Park Avenue South, New York, NY 10010-1710. Tel.: 212-633-3874; Fax: 212-633-3820; E-mail: reprints@elsevier.com.

Clinics in Podiatric Medicine and Surgery is covered in *MEDLINE/PubMed (Index Medicus) and EMBASE/Excerpta Medica.*

Contributors

CONSULTING EDITOR

THOMAS ZGONIS, DPM, FACFAS
Professor and Director, Externship and Reconstructive Foot and Ankle Surgery Fellowship Programs, Division of Podiatric Medicine and Surgery, Department of Orthopaedics, The University of Texas Health Science Center at San Antonio, San Antonio, Texas

EDITOR

ALAN NG, DPM, FACFAS
Residency Committee, PMSR/RRA, Highlands/Presbyterian St. Luke's Podiatric Surgical Residency Program, Private Practice, Advanced Orthopedic and Sports Medicine Specialists, Denver, Colorado

AUTHORS

HANI M. BADAHDAH, DPM, MD, MS
Reconstructive Foot and Ankle Surgery Fellow, Division of Podiatric Medicine and Surgery, Department of Orthopaedics, The University of Texas Health Science Center at San Antonio, San Antonio, Texas

ERIC A. BARP, DPM, FACFAS
Podiatry, The Iowa Clinic, West Des Moines, Iowa

ANDREW BERNHARD, DPM
Attending Physician, PMSR/RRA, Highlands/Presbyterian St. Luke's Podiatric Surgical Residency Program, Denver, Colorado; Private Practice, Eagle-Summit Foot and Ankle, Avon, Colorado

KAITLYN BERNHARD, DPM
Third-Year Resident, PMSR/RRA, Highlands/Presbyterian St. Luke's Podiatric Surgical Residency Program, Denver, Colorado

STEPHEN A. BRIGIDO, DPM, FACFAS
Department Chair and Fellowship Director, Foot and Ankle Reconstruction, Foot and Ankle Department, Coordinated Health, Bethlehem, Pennsylvania

SCOTT C. CARRINGTON, DPM
Associate, American College of Foot and Ankle Surgery, Fellow, Foot and Ankle Reconstruction, Foot and Ankle Department, Coordinated Health, Bethlehem, Pennsylvania

VARUN CHOPRA, DPM
Resident, PMSR/RRA, Highlands/Presbyterian St. Luke's Podiatric Surgical Residency Program, The Colorado Health Foundation, Denver, Colorado

JEFFREY C. CHRISTENSEN, DPM
Podiatric Section, Attending, Department of Orthopedics, Swedish Medical Center, Seattle, Washington; President and Founder, Ankle & Foot Clinics Northwest, Everett, Washington

JOHN G. ERICKSON, DPM
Podiatry, Boone County Hospital, Boone, Iowa

MICHAEL A. GENTILE, DPM, FACFAS
Founding Partner, Northwest Extremity Specialists, Attending Surgeon, Westside Foot and Ankle Specialists, Portland, Oregon

JENNIFER L. HALL, DPM
Podiatric Residency, UnityPoint Health-Des Moines, Des Moines, Iowa

ALEXIS L. KREPLICK, DPM
Resident, PMSR/RRA, West Houston Medical Center, Houston, Texas

MICHAEL S. LEE, DPM, MS, FACFAS
Foot and Ankle Surgery, Capital Orthopaedics and Sports Medicine, PC, Clive, Iowa; Past President, American College of Foot and Ankle Surgeons, Chicago, Illinois

CYNTHIA A. LUU, DPM
Podiatry Resident, Tucson Medical Center, Midwestern University, Tucson, Arizona

SAMUEL S. MENDICINO, DPM, FACFAS
Residency Director, PMSR/RRA, West Houston Medical Center, Houston, Texas

ALAN NG, DPM, FACFAS
Residency Committee, PMSR/RRA, Highlands/Presbyterian St. Luke's Podiatric Surgical Residency Program, Private Practice, Advanced Orthopedic and Sports Medicine Specialists, Denver, Colorado

BENJAMIN D. OVERLEY Jr, DPM, FACFAS
Foot and Ankle Surgery, Coventry Foot and Ankle Surgery, Limerick, Pennsylvania

JASON A. PIRAINO, DPM, MS, FACFAS
Associate Professor, Chief, Foot and Ankle Surgery, Director, Podiatric Medicine and Surgery Residency, Department of Orthopaedics and Rehabilitation, University of Florida College of Medicine – Jacksonville, Jacksonville, Florida

NICOLE M. PROTZMAN, MS
Research Associate, Clinical Integration Department, Coordinated Health, Allentown, Pennsylvania

CHRISTOPHER L. REEVES, DPM, FACFAS
Orlando Foot and Ankle Clinic, Director of Research, Podiatric Surgical Residency Program, Attending Physician, Department of Podiatric Surgery, Florida Hospital East Orlando, Orlando, Florida

MATTHEW R. REMENTER, DPM
Chief Resident, Podiatric Medicine and Surgery Residency, Phoenixville Hospital, Phoenixville, Pennsylvania

JOHN M. SCHUBERTH, DPM
Chief, Foot and Ankle Surgery, Department of Orthopedic Surgery, Kaiser San Francisco Medical Center, Kaiser Foundation Hospital, San Francisco, California

AMBER M. SHANE, DPM, FACFAS
Orlando Foot and Ankle Clinic, Podiatric Surgical Residency Program, Attending Physician, Department of Podiatric Surgery, Florida Hospital East Orlando, Orlando, Florida

JEROME K. STECK, DPM
Southern Arizona Orthopedics, Tucson, Arizona

PAUL STONE, DPM
Program Director, PMSR/RRA, Highlands/Presbyterian St. Luke's Podiatric Surgical Residency Program, The Colorado Health Foundation, Denver, Colorado

RYAN VAZALES, DPM
Residency Training Program, Podiatric Medicine and Surgery, Chief Resident (PGY-3), Florida Hospital East Orlando, Orlando, Florida

JEREMY L. WALTERS, DPM
Sentara Podiatry Specialists, Department of Surgery, Sentara Medical Group, Suffolk, Virginia

THOMAS ZGONIS, DPM, FACFAS
Professor and Director, Externship and Reconstructive Foot and Ankle Surgery Fellowship Programs, Division of Podiatric Medicine and Surgery, Department of Orthopaedics, The University of Texas Health Science Center at San Antonio, San Antonio, Texas

Contents

Nonsurgical treatment of ankle arthritis can be a short-term fix or a long-term solution. An understanding of the biomechanics of the ankle is helpful in the successful use of orthotics and bracing. Pharmacologic and/or biologic treatments can be used exclusively or in concert with mechanical interventions to decrease pain, improve function, and potentially extend the life span of an arthritic ankle.

Ankle arthrodiastasis provides an alternative surgical treatment of the mild to moderate posttraumatic ankle arthritis. Ankle arthrodesis or ankle implant arthroplasty is usually reserved for the end-stage ankle arthritis and after conservative treatment options have been implicated for a long period. Ankle joint destructive procedures are often considered for the older and less active population with strict selected surgical criteria and prolonged rehabilitation. In either ankle joint-sparing or ankle destructive procedures, lower extremity deformity correction will need to be addressed before or at the time of index surgery for the overall patient's successful outcome.

Ankle arthritis can be broadly classified as primary arthritis (nontraumatic degeneration) or secondary arthritis (posttraumatic degeneration). A good understanding of the anatomic features and presentations associated with each will assist the surgeon in determining the best course of action for each patient. Many variations of both primary and secondary arthritis can be treated conservatively; however, there are many times when conservative therapy is not adequate. In these cases, ankle arthroscopy may be considered before a joint fusion or replacement. Here, the authors discuss the common types of ankle arthritis, their presentations, and treatment success with ankle arthroscopy.

Distal tibial malalignment can result from posttraumatic malunion, physeal disturbances, congenital or metabolic diseases, and degenerative arthritis.

Malalignment leads to an altered load distribution across the joint, leading to early ankle joint arthritis. If a substantial part of the joint is salvageable, ankle fusion or joint replacement is not always the best option. Realignment of the distal tibia with a joint-sparing supramalleolar osteotomy is a valuable procedure in correcting deformity at the distal tibia. The goal of a supramalleolar osteotomy is to restore axial alignment. Several studies have demonstrated the successes of the osteotomy in improving function and relieving pain.

Large, symptomatic, focal chondral, and osteochondral lesions of the ankle are treated with osteochondral autograft/allograft transplantation (OAT) procedure, a reconstructive bone grafting technique that uses one or more cylindrical osteochondral grafts from an area of low impact or allograft source and transplants them into the prepared defect site on the talus. This technique allows defects to be filled with mature, hyaline articular cartilage. Acute or chronic chondral or osteochondral lesions can be debilitating; provided here is a review of osteochondral autograft or allograft transplantation. OAT shows a trend toward greater longevity and durability and improved outcomes in high-demand patients.

Repair of osteochondral lesions of the talus can be difficult. Smaller lesions respond well to simple arthroscopy and microfracture, whereas larger cystic lesions may require allograft talus replacement or ankle fusions. The lesions in-between are more difficult to treat. Autologous chondrocyte implantation and matrix-associated autologous chondrocyte implantation have shown promising results. Future research may include new techniques, pharmacologic intervention, and cell-based therapies, and may be better served with prospective observational studies instead of costly randomized controlled studies. A representative example of arthroscopic implantation is given.

First described in 1879, ankle arthrodesis is a procedure that has undergone significant advancements not only in technique but also in technology and fixation. Surgeon preference has often dictated those changes with regard to incisional approaches, fixation methods, and use of bone graft and biologics, but one constant has always remained: open ankle arthrodesis is a predictable, time-tested procedure with consistent results when performed in appropriate patients. This article highlights the changes that have occurred since the introduction of this procedure and provides a brief overview of the preferred technique.

Arthroscopic ankle arthrodesis provides an alternative to open techniques. Advancements in arthroscopic techniques and instrumentation have made the procedure easier to perform. Arthroscopic ankle arthrodesis has demonstrated faster rates of union, fewer complications, reduced postoperative pain, and shorter hospital stays. Sound surgical techniques, particularly with regard to joint preparation, are critical for success. Comorbidities, such as increased body mass index, history of smoking, malalignment, and posttraumatic arthritis should be considered when contemplating arthroscopic ankle arthrodesis. Although total ankle replacement continues to grow in popularity, arthroscopic ankle arthrodesis remains a viable alternative for management of the end-stage arthritic ankle.

Much of the current literature suggests that total ankle replacement (TAR) is no longer an inferior or fringe treatment for advanced ankle arthritis compared with ankle fusion, but rather a viable option for recalcitrant arthritic ankle pathology in the correct patient population. In this article, current concepts associated with successful outcomes for TAR are discussed with an emphasis on ankle joint anatomy and biomechanics, preoperative planning and patient selection, understanding pathomechanics and soft tissue balancing, as well as the surgeon's learning curve.

Total ankle arthroplasty is a viable surgical technique for the treatment of end-stage degenerative joint disease. With continued advancement in prosthetic design, refined surgical techniques, and improved outcomes, the indications for total ankle replacement have expanded to include cases of increasing complexity. With meticulous preoperative planning and exacting execution, many frontal plane deformities and cases of avascular necrosis can now be successfully addressed at the time of prosthesis implantation or in a staged procedure.

With total ankle arthroplasty, documented complications can be categorized chronologically into intraoperative, postoperative, and late complications. Factors such as patient selection, surgeon experience, implant features, and prosthetic device selection can influence functional outcomes as well as incidence of complications. Even with impeccable surgical technique and optimal patient selection, complications that require revision may still arise. The most common complications with revision solutions are discussed in this article.

Total ankle arthroplasty (TAA) and ankle arthrodesis (AA) are complicated surgeries that carry a learning curve. Complications are an aspect of all surgeries that must be considered. Surgeons must be prepared to handle these complications. The most important things are early identification and treatment of these complications. Treating complications is a combination of medicines, conservative measures, and, most importantly, surgical intervention. Recent studies have shown a decrease in complications of TAA and AA over the past 10 years. Carefully identifying the complications early and treating patients right away are imperative to improving the outcomes for these patients.

CLINICS IN PODIATRIC MEDICINE AND SURGERY

RELATED INTEREST

Foot and Ankle Clinics, June 2017 (Vol. 22, Issue 2)
Current Updates in Total Ankle Arthroplasty
J. Chris Coetzee, *Editor*
Available at: http://www.foot.theclinics.com/

THE CLINICS ARE AVAILABLE ONLINE!
Access your subscription at:
www.theclinics.com

Preface

The Evolution of Arthritis Treatment in the Foot and Ankle: A Change in the Gold Standard?

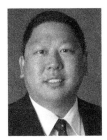

Alan Ng, DPM, FACFAS
Editor

It's amazing when we look back over the past ten years and evaluate how we treated ankle arthritis then and how we treat arthritis now. The combinations of new techniques and new technology have changed the way we evaluate and treat ankle arthritis. Ten years ago, ankle arthrodesis was considered the "gold standard" for degenerative arthritis of the ankle. Today we are seeing more and more total ankle arthroplasties being performed and are now questioning if total ankle arthroplasty is becoming the "gold standard." Development of new technology has us reevaluating how we treat injuries to the articular cartilage where in the past we would excise and perform some type of marrow stimulation and hope that arthritis would not develop until later in life. Treatment of osteochondral lesions of the ankle has advanced over the past 10 years with new techniques that have relied on improved grafting techniques and development of different allografts and synthetic materials to assist in regenerating hyaline-like cartilage. New thought processes and looking at the lower extremity as a whole have resulted in better long-term patient outcomes. Advanced techniques with evaluation of pertinent angles and alignment of the entire extremity and not just the ankle joint have allowed us to prolong the need for joint destructive procedures. The foot and ankle surgeon must understand and evaluate new advances in surgical technique and decide if it is a viable option for their practice. Many procedures have stood the test of time and are discussed in this *Clinics in Podiatric Medicine and Surgery* issue. Ankle arthrodesis has been a successful procedure and has stood the test of time; we discuss new approaches and concepts in ankle arthrodesis. Total ankle arthroplasty has been proven to be a successful procedure, but proper evaluation and criteria should be followed if the foot and ankle surgeon is planning to add this procedure to their practice. Understanding risk factors, patient comorbidities, and alignment is

Clin Podiatr Med Surg 34 (2017) xv–xvi
http://dx.doi.org/10.1016/j.cpm.2017.07.001
0891-8422/17/© 2017 Published by Elsevier Inc.

crucial to successful outcomes. We have dedicated a significant portion of this *Clinics in Podiatric Medicine and Surgery* issue to dealing with complications and revision techniques for Total Ankle Arthroplasty. As we see this procedure becoming more mainstream, we will see an increase in failures, which will need revision surgery or conversion to complex ankle arthrodesis.

We are living in an exciting time of technology and advances in surgical techniques. I can only imagine what is on the horizon for treatment of arthritis; 10 years from now techniques and technology will be developed that will change the entire landscape of foot and ankle surgery.

Authors of the following articles are leaders in the field and current subject matter experts in treatment of ankle arthritis. I would like to thank them for their contribution to this *Clinics in Podiatric Medicine and Surgery* issue and hope that the following articles will assist the foot and ankle surgeon in treatment of ankle arthritis.

Alan Ng, DPM, FACFAS
Advanced Orthopedic and Sports Medicine Specialists
8101 East Lowry Boulevard, #230
Denver, CO 80230, USA

E-mail address:
ankleftdoc@aol.com

Nonsurgical Treatment of Ankle Arthritis

Michael A. Gentile, DPM

KEYWORDS

- Conservative • Nonsurgical • Ankle arthritis • Ankle bracing

KEY POINTS

- Nonsurgical care of ankle arthritis can be remarkably successful. A firm understanding of the options available, either alone or in combination, is beneficial.
- Applying knowledge of the 3 intervals of the stance phase of gait may lead to better outcomes with bracing. Understanding the apex and flexibility of deformity may improve patient tolerance.
- Injectable steroids can provide good pain relief if used thoughtfully. Confirmation of needle placement is helpful to better understanding of the success or failure of these injections.
- The use of biologic options, such as platelet-rich plasma (PRP), amnion, or stem cells, provides the potential for preservation and/or regeneration of the joint. Early data are encouraging.

INTRODUCTION

Bipedal locomotion is a gift and an affliction for the human race. When the ankle is fully loaded at 500 N, the total contact area is 350 mm^2.[1,2] This is compared with 1120 mm^2 for the knee[3] and 1100 mm^2 for the hip.[3] Even though the cartilage in the hip and knee is thicker, the articular cartilage of the ankle shows greater tensile strength over a longer period of time. This may explain the relative resistance of the ankle to increasing arthritis with age compared with the hip and knee.[4,5]

Ankle arthritis has a significant impact on quality of life. Using the 36-Item Short Form Health Survey (SF-36), Glazebrook and colleagues[6] found similar scores between patients with end-stage ankle versus hip arthritis. Agel and colleagues[7] found that patients with end-stage ankle arthritis scored 3 times worse than normal patients using the Musculoskeletal Functional Assessment. Segal and colleagues[8] correlated SF-36 and Musculoskeletal Functional Assessment scores to gait kinematics and step count. They found those with ankle arthritis had lower scores,

Disclosure Statement: None.
Northwest Extremity Specialists, Westside Foot and Ankle Specialists, 9900 Southwest Hall Boulevard, Suite 100, Portland, OR 97223, USA
E-mail address: ahinga74@gmail.com

Clin Podiatr Med Surg 34 (2017) 415–423
http://dx.doi.org/10.1016/j.cpm.2017.06.001
0891-8422/17/© 2017 Elsevier Inc. All rights reserved.

reduced ankle range of motion, peak ankle power absorbed, and peak ankle power generated.

Nonsurgical or conservative care is at times considered an obligatory step on the road to surgery. In some cases it may be enough to provide patients the quality of life and function they deserve and desire. For other patients, it may be the only option. Examples include personal choice, age, occupation or desired activities, confluence of comorbidities, or a history of infection. In these situations, a surgeon should be well versed with the options available.

This article explores the nonsurgical options available for ankle arthritis. These options can be categorized as mechanical, pharmacologic, and regenerative/restorative. When possible, an evidence-based evaluation is provided. Indications, appropriateness, and expectations are reviewed.

BIOMECHANICS OF THE ANKLE JOINT

Gait can be divided into stance and swing phases. Comprising 62% of the total gait cycle, stance is further divided into 3 intervals. The effects on the ankle joint are highlighted.

First Interval: Heel Strike Until Foot Is Flat on the Ground

- Foot absorbs and dissipates the forces generated from the foot contacting the ground.
- Primarily a passive event governed by the mobility of the subtalar joint and translated distally into the midtarsal joint complex.
- The initial contact with the ground and the shift of the body's center of gravity generate a vertical force concentration of 15% to 25% of body weight.
- Ankle undergoes marked plantarflexion.

Second Interval: Foot Flat on the Ground to Early Heel Lift

- Foot begins transition from mobile adapter to more rigid lever.
- Dynamic input from extrinsic muscles and continued translation through leg, subtalar, and midtarsal joints.
- Ankle reaches maximum dorsiflexion and force concentration of 4.5 times body weight. It is during dorsiflexion that the ankle has its greatest contact area.

Third Interval: Heel Lift Through Toe-off

- Foot becomes more rigid.
- Continued dynamic input from extrinsic musculature, which includes the triceps surae, creating active ankle plantarflexion.
- Continued ankle plantarflexion is due to momentum.

MECHANICAL INTERVENTIONS

Controlling or manipulating the forces through the ankle joint may seem at first a simple concept. It is, however, more than just limiting motion in the ankle. Applying an understanding of the stance phase of gait and precisely where in this phase the patient is most symptomatic results in greater success. Torsional issues and malalignment proximal to the ankle change the contact area as well as the characteristics and intensity of the forces within the joint. Limited subtalar and/or midtarsal joint motion negate force dissipation and translation and focus it within the ankle.

Foot Orthotics

The simplest option is the use of a functional orthotic. Expectations of an orthotic include

- Shifting the contact point and thus loading pressures within the ankle
- Slowing the velocity of the foot as it goes from the first to second interval of stance
- Correcting malalignment of the hindfoot

Treatment success is directly proportional to the flexibility along the entirety of the kinetic chain but especially the foot. A rigid deformity is not likely to be amenable to a foot orthotic and frankly may cause more pain and functional decline. In this case, an accommodative orthotic may be more appropriate to provide improved shock absorption and force dissipation, in other words, making the foot more comfortable where it is.

Bracing

Bracing is indicated in situations where an orthotic has failed or is not appropriate. Indications for bracing include

- Rigid foot deformity with a supple ankle
- Frontal plane deformity in the ankle or suprapedal deformity with a flexible foot and ankle
- Patients who are not surgical candidates for whom the goal is to spread weight-bearing forces over the largest surface area possible

If a deformity cannot be manually reduced, plastic and leather cannot be expected to be successful. The goal, however, may not be deformity correction but simply symptom relief. In this situation, an attempt at bracing may be reasonable. This may be further enabled by incorporating a foot orthotic into the brace.

Off-the-shelf bracing is convenient. It is also a litmus test for a patients' tolerance to custom bracing and may soften them to the idea that bracing can be successful. The greater the stability of the brace, the more the motion in the ankle is limited. Furthermore, edema can be problematic in these patients and the compression afforded by the brace may be an additional benefit. In cases of severe edema, difficulty with donning the brace or intolerance to circumferential brace contact, a carbon ToeOFF AFO may be remarkably useful (**Fig. 1**).

Custom braces can either hinged (with or without lock-outs) or locked, short or long. A more anatomic contour to the posterior musculature can possibly provide more effective offloading. Expectations should be tempered with significant frontal plane deformities with boney prominences or rigid deformities. Bracing may be intolerable despite multiple attempts at accommodation.

Hinged braces can be useful in patients who have more proximal pathology where force and stress migration would create new or increased pain. The ability to control how much motion is available can help in finding the sweet spot or, if this does not happen, the lock-out can be used and brace made rigid. Unfortunately, a brace can only be successful if a patient uses it.

PHARMACOLOGIC INTERVENTION

Aside from the standard recommendations of over-the-counter medications, such as acetaminophen and/or nonsteroidal anti-inflammatories, other options are available.

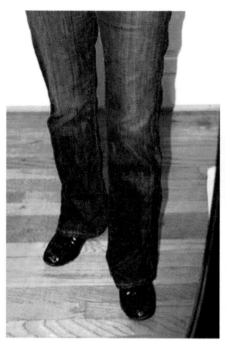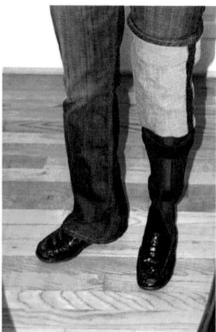

Fig. 1. Example of a ToeOFF AFO. These braces are low profile and fit easily into a variety of shoes.

Injectable Steroid Therapy

The use of injectable steroids can prove useful for symptom relief. The use of an acetate-based injectable can be controversial with the fear that the injectable itself can further progress soft tissue and/or cartilage degeneration. If the ankle is beyond salvage, however, the risk to benefit ratio may make sense. In the author's experience, a steroid injection is most useful if there is some level of inflammation in the ankle. If the first injection fails to provide significant pain relief, a repeat injection may be of little to no value unless there is image-guided needle placement. Ultrasound or fluoroscopy provides objective evidence that the needle was placed into the ankle as intended (**Fig. 2**). The following is the author's preferred technique (**Fig. 3**):

- Iodine prep to the anterior medial shoulder
    - Measured 1 cm from tip of the medial malleolus and just medial to the tibialis anterior tendon
- With the ankle in dorsiflexion to protect the talar articular surface, the needle is directed approximately 45° lateral and into anterior capsular pouch.
- Preferred medication cocktail
    - 2 mL 0.5% bupivacaine with epinephrine
    - 1 mL betamethasone sodium phosphate/betamethasone acetate (30 mg/5 mL)

Viscosupplementation has been used with some success. Unfortunately use in the ankle is considered off-label and thus insurance coverage is unlikely. Data suggest that the improvement in functional scores is at least comparable to saline placebo. The upside is there are no reported significant adverse events.[9–14] The

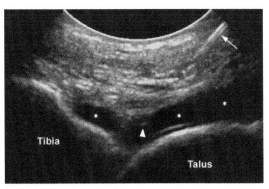

Fig. 2. Long-axis image of ultrasound-guided ankle injection. The arrow represents the needle prior to being introduced into the anterior capsular pouch (*arrowhead*, joint capsule; *asterisk*, anterior pouch).

rationale behind its use is to increase the shock absorption qualities of the joint fluid, dulling of intracapsular nociceptors, and perhaps an increase synovial fluid production.

REGENERATIVE OR BIOLOGIC INTERVENTION

So-called biologic or regenerative interventions are gaining popularity. Amniotic fluid and PRP both aim to deliver a concentrate of growth factors and essentially relieve pain and improve function. Stem cell therapy provides the potential for actual regeneration and maintenance of articular-like cartilage.

Platelet-Rich Plasma

PRP is gaining popularity in both the nonsurgical and surgical treatment of focal osteochondral defects (OCDs) and global arthritis. Data suggest that a leukocyte-poor product may have fewer proinflammatory effects and less collagen breakdown (including cartilage) due to fewer metalloproteinases.[15]

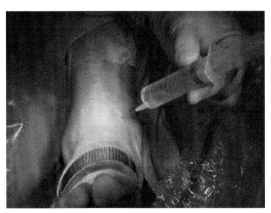

Fig. 3. Preferred method of ankle injection. Needle is introduced at the medial shoulder, just medial to the tibialis anterior tendon. Needle is angled at approximately 45° to avoid inadvertent cartilage damage.

Current data suggest the following effects in cell cultures:

- Increased chondrocyte proliferation rate, phenotype expression, and maintenance[16-19]
- Increased matrix molecule production[16-19]
- Increased expression of type II collagen[16,20]
- Enhanced expression, chondrocyte differentiation, migration, and adhesion of mesenchymal stem cells[16,20,21]
- Potential anti-inflammatory effects (if leukocyte poor)[16-19,22]

Animal study data are more mixed and differ between OCDs and general osteoarthritis (OA). In a rat model, there were conflicting data.[23] In a rabbit model, there was a positive influence on cartilage degeneration. In a pig rheumatoid arthritis model, there was diminished inflammation and a chondroprotective effect.[24-26]

Clinical studies have been extrapolated from the knee. In 1 randomized control trial on talar OCDs, Mei-Dan and colleagues[27] showed statistically significant improvement in clinical scores compared with hyaluronic acid with 7 months' mean follow-up. In the only global ankle OA trial, Angthong and colleagues[28] demonstrated significant clinical improvement but no change in OA grade on MRI at 16 months. Mei-Dan and colleagues, however, provided a 2-times to 3-times basal rate cell concentration versus low platelet count in the other study. Both used leukocyte poor injectates. This suggests that the concentration of available cells is directly correlated with biologic effect.

Amnion Injections

Micronized dehydrated human amnion/chorion membrane injections are also garnering interest. As with PRP, there is not enough evidence to make definitive recommendations. In 2 OA-induced rat models, cartilage degeneration was attenuated versus control.[29,30] There seemed to be a potential dose-dependent effect with greater benefit at 4 weeks postinjection with a higher concentration of injectate.[29]

Newly available fresh, nondehydrated amnion grafts have been shown to include live cells. If these cells are confirmed to be viable pluripotent mesenchymal stem cells, there is the promise of possible chondrogenic properties. In addition, these grafts have been shown to maintain their native structure, including an intact and open extracellular matrix. This is thought to provide an improved scaffold for tissue growth and thus improved integration to the recipient tissue.

Stem Cell Therapy

The new frontier of cartilage repair seems to be in stem cell therapy. Whether derived from adipose tissue or bone marrow stromal cells, there are early data suggesting the following benefits[31]:

- Decreased intra-articular inflammation and enhanced immunomodulation
- Increased cartilage production
- Decreased native cartilage degeneration

The challenges lie in confirming the reliable potential of the stem cells to differentiate into chondrocytes and to produce a native and structural functional unit. Protocols differ on whether the stem cells should be used alone or combined with PRP and an extracellular matrix to expand and activate the stem cells while providing a scaffold for growth.

Jo and colleagues[32] have shown the greatest promise with adipose-derived stem cells (ADSCs). In a randomized double-blind study, they used MRI and arthroscopy to show the regeneration of articular-like cartilage. High-dose ADSCs (100 million) were shown more efficacious. Furthermore, they used only autologous culture expanded cells without PRP or extracellular matrix. Other studies by Koh and colleagues[33] and Kim and colleagues[34] have shown that with lower numbers of ADSCs, use of PRP or fibrin glue improves functional scores. Second-look arthroscopy, however, showed fibrocartilage instead of hyaline-like cartilage.

DISCUSSION

Patients with ankle arthritis have a host of nonsurgical treatments available. Whether used as a long-term solution or a short-term fix, a firm understanding of the rationale of each treatment option will likely lead to greater pain relief and increased or at least maintained function. In the end, a logical combination of mechanical, pharmacologic, and biologic customized to each patient should be considered. Although regenerative medicine shows promise, there are not enough quality data to make specific treatment recommendations.

REFERENCES

1. Beaudoin AJ, Fiore SM, Krause WR, et al. Effect of isolated talocalcaneal fusion on contact in the ankle and talonavicular joints. Foot Ankle 1991;12:19–25.
2. Kimizuka M, Kurosawa H, Fukubayashi T. Load-bearing pattern of the ankle joint. Contact area and pressure distribution. Arch Orthop Trauma Surg 1980;96:45–9.
3. Ihn JC, Kim SJ, Park IH. In vitro study of contact area and pressure distribution in the human knee after partial and total meniscectomy. Int Orthop 1993;17:214–8.
4. Brown TD, Shaw DT. In vitro contact stress distributions in the natural human hip. J Biomech 1983;16:373–84.
5. Kempson GE. Age-related changes in the tensile properties of human articular cartilage: a comparative study between the femoral head of the hip joint and the talus of the ankle joint. Biochim Biophys Acta 1991;1075:223–30.
6. Glazebrook M, Daniels T, Younger A, et al. Comparison of health-related quality of life between patients with end-stage ankle and hip arthrosis. J Bone Joint Surg Am 2008;90:499–505.
7. Agel J, Coetzee JC, Sangeorzan BJ, et al. Functional limitations of patients with end-stage ankle arthrosis. Foot Ankle Int 2005;26:537–9.
8. Segal AD, Shofer J, Hahn ME, et al. Functional limitations associated with end-stage ankle arthritis. J Bone Joint Surg Am 2012;94:777–83.
9. Cohen MM, Altman RD, Hollstrom R, et al. Safety and efficacy of intra-articular sodium hyaluronate (Hyalgan) in a randomized, double-blind study for osteoarthritis of the ankle. Foot Ankle Int 2008;29:657–63.
10. DeGroot H 3rd, Uzunishvili S, Weir R, et al. Intra-articular injection of hyaluronic acid is not superior to saline solution injection for ankle arthritis: a randomized, double-blind, placebo-controlled study. J Bone Joint Surg Am 2012;94:2–8.
11. Salk RS, Chang TJ, D'Costa WF, et al. Sodium hyaluronate in the treatment of osteoarthritis of the ankle: a controlled, randomized, double-blind pilot study. J Bone Joint Surg Am 2006;88:295–302.
12. Sun SF, Chou YJ, Hsu CW, et al. Efficacy of intra-articular hyaluronic acid in patients with osteoarthritis of the ankle: a prospective study. Osteoarthritis Cartilage 2006;14:867–74.
13. Sun SF, Hsu CW, Sun HP, et al. The effect of three weekly intra-articular injections of hyaluronate on pain, function, and balance in patients with unilateral ankle arthritis. J Bone Joint Surg Am 2011;93:1720–6.

14. Witteveen AG, Sierevelt IN, Blankevoort L, et al. Intra-articular sodium hyaluronate injections in the osteoarthritic ankle joint: effects, safety and dose dependency. Foot Ankle Surg 2010;16:159–63.
15. Vannini F, Di Mateo B, Filardo G. Platelet-rich plasma to treat ankle cartilage pathology-From translational potential to clinical evidence: a systematic review. J Exp Orthop 2015;2(1):2.
16. Filardo G, Kon E, Roffi A, et al. Platelet-rich plasma: why intra-articular? A systematic review of preclinical studies and clinical evidence on PRP for joint degeneration. Knee Surg Sports Traumatol Arthrosc 2013;23(9):2459–74.
17. Muraglia A, Ottonello C, Spanò R, et al. Biological activity of a standardized freeze-dried platelet derivative to be used as cell culture medium supplement. Platelets 2014;25(3):211–20.
18. Park SI, Lee HR, Kim S, et al. Time-sequential modulation in expression of growth factors from platelet-rich plasma (PRP) on the chondrocyte cultures. Mol Cell Biochem 2012;361(1–2):9–17.
19. Lee HR, Park KM, Joung YK, et al. Platelet- rich plasma loaded hydrogel scaffold enhances chondrogenic differentiation and maturation with up-regulation of CB1 and CB2. J Control Release 2012;159(3):332–7.
20. Mifune Y, Matsumoto T, Takayama K, et al. The effect of platelet-rich plasma on the regenerative therapy of muscle derived stem cells for articular cartilage repair. Osteoarthritis Cartil 2013;21(1):175–85.
21. Hildner F, Eder MJ, Hofer K, et al. Human platelet lysate successfully promotes proliferation and subsequent chondrogenic differentiation of adipose-derived stem cells: a comparison with articular chondrocytes. J Tissue Eng Regen Med 2015;9(7):808–18.
22. Assirelli E, Filardo G, Mariani E, et al. Effect of two different preparations of platelet-rich plasma on synoviocytes. Knee Surg Sports Traumatol Arthrosc 2015;23(9):2690–703.
23. Guner S, Buyukbebeci O. Analyzing the effects of platelet gel on knee osteoarthritis in the rat model. Clin Appl Thromb Hemost 2013;19(5):494–8.
24. Kwon DR, Park GY, Lee SU. The effects of intra-articular platelet-rich plasma injection according to the severity of collagenase-induced knee osteoarthritis in a rabbit model. Ann Rehabil Med 2012;36(4):458–65.
25. Saito M, Takahashi KA, Arai Y, et al. Intraarticular administration of platelet-rich plasma with biodegradable gelatin hydrogel microspheres prevents osteoarthritis progression in the rabbit knee. Clin Exp Rheumatol 2009;27(2):201–7.
26. Serra CI, Soler C, Carillo JM, et al. Effect of autologous platelet-rich plasma on the repair of full-thickness articular defects in rabbits. Knee Surg Sports Traumatol Arthrosc 2013;21(8):1730–6.
27. Mei-Dan O, Carmont MR, Laver L, et al. Platelet-rich plasma or hyaluronate in the management of osteochondral lesions of the talus. Am J Sports Med 2012;40(3):534–41.
28. Angthong C, Khadsongkram A, Angthong W. Outcomes and quality of life after platelet-rich plasma therapy in patients with recalcitrant hindfoot and ankle diseases: a preliminary report of 12 patients. J Foot Ankle Surg 2013;52(4):475–80.
29. Raines A, Shih MS, Chua L, et al. Efficacy of particulate amniontic membrane and umbilical cord tissues in attenuating cartilage destruction in an osteoarthritis model. Tissue Eng A 2017;23(1–2):12–9.
30. Willett NJ, Thote T, Lin AS, et al. Intra-articular injection of micronized dehydrated human amnion/chorion membrane attenuates osteoarthritis development. Arthritis Res Ther 2014;16(1):R472014, 16(1): R47.

31. Pak J, Lee JH, Kartolo WA, et al. Cartilage regeneration in humans with adipose tissue-derived stem cells: current status in clinical implications. Biomed Res Int 2016;2016:4702674.
32. Jo CH, Lee YG, Shin WH, et al. Intra-articular injection of mesenchymal stem cells for the treatment of osteoarthritis of the knee: a proof-of-concept clinical trial. Stem Cells 2014;32(5):1254–66.
33. Koh YG, Choi YJ, Kwon OR, et al. Second-look arthroscopic evaluation of cartilage lesions after mesenchymal stem cell implantation in osteoarthritic knees. Am J Sports Med 2014;42(7):1628–37.
34. Kim YS, Choi YJ, Suh DS, et al. Mesenchymal stem cell implantation in osteoarthritic knees: is fibrin glue effective as a scaffold? Am J Sports Med 2015;43(1): 176–85.

Ankle Arthrodiastasis with Circular External Fixation for the Treatment of Posttraumatic Ankle Arthritis

Hani M. Badahdah, DPM, MD, MS, Thomas Zgonis, DPM*

KEYWORDS

- External fixation • Ankle arthrodiastasis • Distraction • Surgery
- Posttraumatic arthritis

KEY POINTS

- Ankle arthrodiastasis is indicated in the younger and active population.
- Ankle arthrodesis or ankle implant arthroplasty is usually reserved for the end-stage ankle arthritis.
- Concomitant osseous and soft tissues procedures are highly recommended to be performed before or at the same time of ankle arthrodiastasis.

INTRODUCTION

Posttraumatic arthritis of the ankle is a challenging pathologic entity for the treating physician and surgeon. As primary osteoarthritis is more common in the hip and knee joints, posttraumatic arthritis is found mostly in the ankle joint and is one of the main reasons for surgical intervention.[1] Posttraumatic ankle arthritis presents a unique challenge in the juvenile or younger and active population with or without the presence of a lower extremity deformity.[2–4] Ankle destructive procedures such as ankle arthrodesis or ankle implant arthroplasty are usually reserved for the older and less active population without any significant medical comorbidities.

Ankle arthrodesis is a joint destructive procedure and is considered by many investigators the gold standard for the end-stage posttraumatic ankle arthritis. In 2015, a retrospective study by Kawoosa and colleagues[5] studied the use of circular external fixation for a primary or revisional ankle arthrodesis in various ankle abnormalities. In their study, all 16 patients had a successful ankle union at an average of 14 weeks.

Disclosure: The authors have nothing to disclose.
Division of Podiatric Medicine and Surgery, Department of Orthopaedics, The University of Texas Health Science Center at San Antonio, 7703 Floyd Curl Drive, MSC 7776, San Antonio, TX 78229, USA
* Corresponding author.
E-mail address: zgonis@uthscsa.edu

In another retrospective study by Mongon and colleagues,[6] all 17 patients with ankle arthrodesis for posttraumatic arthritis had an ankle union at an average of 16.6 weeks. In 2012, Gowda and Kumar[7] have shown successful ankle arthrodesis results in all 15 patients with posttraumatic arthritis by using the Charnley's external fixation system. The use of Taylor spatial frame for ankle arthrodesis in various ankle abnormalities was also studied by Thiryayi and colleagues,[8] where they found successful union in all of their 10 patients. However, long-term sequelae of ankle arthrodesis may include and are not limited to functional limitation, overload of the adjacent and contralateral foot and ankle joints with potential development of joint arthritis, nonunion, malunion, and infection, which usually will require a revisional surgery.

Ankle implant arthroplasty is an alternative to ankle arthrodesis with selective surgical criteria. Older patients without significant medical comorbidities, average body mass index, and low activity level with minimal or absent lower extremity deformity represent the ideal group for the ankle implant arthroplasty procedure.[3,9] Intermediate to long-term outcomes of 82 patients by using the Scandinavian Total Ankle Replacement by Nunley and colleagues[10] showed satisfactory results in improving the patient's function and quality of life while decreasing the level of pain. In another study by Saltzman and colleagues,[11] a comparison of early outcomes between an ankle arthrodesis and ankle implant arthroplasty of 138 patients showed similar results for an average follow-up of 4 years. In the same study, more complications that required surgical intervention were noted in the ankle implant arthroplasty group. In addition, Ellington and colleagues[12] in a retrospective study of 53 patients with a failed Agility total ankle implant have concluded that a revisional ankle implant arthroplasty may be considered instead of an ankle arthrodesis when dealing with failure of this particular ankle implant.

In lieu of the above potential devastating complications and strict selective surgical criteria with an ankle arthrodesis or ankle implant arthroplasty, ankle arthrodiastasis is a joint-sparing procedure that provides an alternative option for the treatment of posttraumatic ankle arthritis. Current literature has shown that ankle arthrodiastasis can relieve the patient's pain, improve function, and delay or exclude the need for the ankle joint destructive procedures.[9]

Paley and colleagues[13] in a review of 32 patients with ankle arthrodiastasis and concomitant osseous and soft tissue procedures found that 78% of their patients had satisfactory results maintaining their ankle range of motion. Zgonis and colleagues[14] have described the technique of a simultaneous ankle arthrodiastasis and subtalar joint arthrodesis for posttraumatic arthrosis, whereas Ramanujam and colleagues[15] described this technique with the addition of a talar dome resurfacing with the use of a collagen-glycosaminoglycan monolayer. Fragomen and colleagues[16] suggested that 5 mm of ankle arthrodiastasis was not enough to prevent contact of the ankle articular surfaces during weight-bearing in a cadaveric study of 9 specimens. However, a retrospective study of 29 patients by Nguyen and colleagues[17] found that ankle function had declined over time in patients with ankle arthrodiastasis for the treatment of end-stage osteoarthritis.

ANKLE ARTHRODIASTASIS

Arthrodiastasis promotes an optimal environment for cartilage repair through mechanical unloading of the ankle joint and restoration of intermittent intra-articular hydrostatic pressure.[18] Unloading the periarticular subchondral bone with ankle arthrodiastasis is an additional mechanism leading to cartilage repair. This continuous reparative process may interrupt the progression and deterioration of the ankle joint articular cartilage.[2,18]

Concomitant osseous and soft tissues procedures are highly recommended to be performed before or at the same time of the ankle arthrodiastasis procedure. For example, lower extremity osseous deformities can be addressed with a simultaneous supramalleolar, fibular or calcaneal osteotomy, and/or subtalar joint arthrodesis or subtalar joint arthrodiastasis when indicated. In addition, talar subchondral drilling, cartilage transplantation, talar resurfacing with orthobiologics at the time of open ankle arthrotomy and/or exostectomy, or application of mesenchymal stem cells[18] can also be added to the ankle arthrodiastasis procedure. Similarly, ankle and periarticular soft tissue releases, synovectomies, and equinus correction with gastrocnemius recession or tendo-Achilles lengthening might also be necessary at the time of ankle arthrodiastasis.

Preoperative planning is a critical step in the selection criteria process of patients who would benefit from an ankle arthrodiastasis procedure. A thorough history and physical examination should include the patient's age, activity level, tobacco use, alcohol abuse, social support, medical comorbidities, history of osseous or ligamentous ankle or lower extremity injuries, retained hardware, previous history of osteomyelitis or open wounds, presence of neuropathy, open fractures, or compartment syndrome.

Lower extremity neurovascular status, ankle joint range of motion, equinus deformity, ankle instability, and/or deformity should be included and documented during the physical examination. Weight-bearing foot, calcaneal, ankle, tibia-fibula or further proximal radiographs, gait analysis, and medical imaging such as computed tomography or MRI are strongly recommended for thorough evaluation of the ankle joint and ligamentous structures.[9] In addition, a thorough discussion with the patient about the surgical procedure, external fixation device, weight-bearing status, postoperative course, pain management, potential complications, rehabilitation, and surgical expectations is beneficial for the patient's successful recovery.

Patients with peripheral vascular disease, infection, Charcot neuroarthropathy, dense peripheral neuropathy, and noncompliance are some of the major contraindications for an ankle arthrodiastasis procedure. Relative contraindications may include and are not limited to patients with active smoking, alcohol abuse, uncontrolled diabetes mellitus, lymphedema and venous insufficiency, previous or current history of compartment syndrome, severe arthritic changes of the ankle joint, and morbid obesity.[2,9,19]

SURGICAL TIPS AND PEARLS

Ankle arthrodiastasis with circular external fixation is performed under regional or general anesthesia with the patient placed in the supine position. Pneumatic tourniquet use is highly recommended during the procedure, which is deflated before the application of the circular external fixation device. An anteromedial ankle incision is made just medial to the tibialis anterior tendon, avoiding any major neurovascular structures. Next, an open ankle arthrotomy with synovectomy and soft tissue release is made, and any osteophytes or loose bodies are removed from the ankle joint. Ankle range of motion is assessed, and if it is still limited in the absence of an osseous block, an open or percutaneous gastrocnemius recession or tendo-Achilles lengthening is then performed. At that time, talar subchondral drilling, cartilage microfracture, or transplantation and/or talar resurfacing with orthobiologics might be performed. Next, all surgical incisions are closed, and the tourniquet is then deflated.

The circular external fixation is applied in a percutaneous fashion, and ankle arthrodiastasis is achieved under direct visualization with an intraoperative C-arm fluoroscopic imaging. Most common circular external fixation devices for this technique comprise 2 tibial rings connected to a foot plate or a midfoot ring with ankle hinges, threaded rods, or struts to aid in the acute or gradual ankle arthrodiastasis procedure. If an isolated ankle arthrodiastasis is performed, talar fixation is secured to the foot plate or midfoot ring. Other types of circular external fixation devices are based on computer programs and can provide the necessary symmetric arthrodiastasis by the utilization of struts connecting the tibial rings to the foot plate or midfoot ring. It has been recommended that 5- to 10-mm acute axial ankle arthrodiastasis can be accomplished intraoperatively, which can also be performed gradually postoperatively.[9,19,20] In many cases, a simultaneous subtalar joint arthrodiastasis can be performed if indicated. For those cases of a simultaneous ankle and subtalar joint arthrodiastasis, no talar fixation is secured to the foot plate or midfoot ring, and the procedure is performed by the necessary ankle hinges, threaded rods, or struts depending on the circular external fixation device (**Fig. 1**).

In contrast, in the presence of any osseous deformities proximal or distal to the ankle joint level, ankle arthrodiastasis is performed after the osseous deformity correction and alignment. For example, a supramalleolar or calcaneal osteotomy and/or subtalar joint arthrodesis might be necessary to be performed before the ankle arthrodiastasis procedure and circular external fixation application.

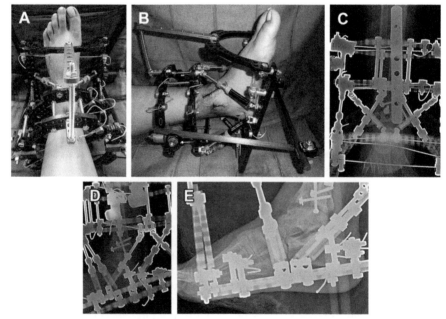

Fig. 1. Postoperative clinical (*A, B*) and radiographic (*C–E*) views showing a simultaneous ankle and subtalar joint arthrodiastasis with an open ankle arthrotomy, exostectomy, and removal of one painful medial malleolus screw in a young patient with posttraumatic ankle arthritis. Note the symmetric ankle (*D*) and simultaneous subtalar joint arthrodiastasis (*E*) without any talar fixation secured to the foot plate of the Taylor spatial frame. The modified "kickstand" apparatus at the inferior aspect of the external fixation foot plate (*B*) can be removed at any time during the postoperative course if partial or full weight-bearing is desired.

POSTOPERATIVE COURSE

The patient's postoperative course is dependent on the concomitant procedures performed with the ankle arthrodiastasis. If no osseous procedures are performed, the patient may be allowed to a full-weight-bearing status within 10 to 14 days after the initial surgery. Necessary gradual ankle arthrodiastasis is performed during the outpatient clinic visits and serial radiographs of the lower extremity. However, in the presence of simultaneous osseous procedures at the time of ankle arthrodiastasis, full weight-bearing status might be delayed, whereas the duration of the circular external fixation device might also be prolonged during the postoperative course. For an isolated ankle arthrodiastasis procedure, an average of 10 ± 2 weeks duration of the circular external fixation device is recommended depending on the severity of ankle arthritis and acute or gradual arthrodiastasis technique, although other investigators have reported on removal of the circular external fixation at earlier times.[20]

A prospective comparative study of ankle arthrodiastasis in a younger population by Herrera-Pérez and colleagues[21] showed that ankle arthrodiastasis was superior to an isolated ankle synovectomy for the treatment of posttraumatic ankle arthritis. In this study,[21] the investigators used a unilateral external fixation device, which was maintained for at least 3 months. In another study by van Valburg and colleagues,[22] an average of 3 months arthrodiastasis was maintained with the circular external fixation device as it was also reported in an open prospective and randomized controlled study by Marijnissen and colleagues.[23] Furthermore, in a study by Ploegmakers and colleagues[24] on the prolonged clinical benefits of ankle arthrodiastasis for the treatment of ankle osteoarthritis, the circular external fixation was maintained for an average of 15 ± 3 weeks.

After removal of the external fixation device, the patient may be progressed to a walking cast, boot, or normal supportive shoe gear with physical therapy and rehabilitation if needed. Patients may return to full activity level at approximately 3 to 4 months postoperatively.[9,18,25]

SUMMARY

Posttraumatic ankle arthritis is a challenging and disabling disorder that affects primarily younger patients. Ankle arthrodiastasis is a promising procedure that offers alternative options to ankle destructive procedures. Concomitant soft tissue and osseous procedures might need to be addressed at the time of ankle arthrodiastasis. Further higher levels of evidence studies are required to address the efficacy and long-term outcomes of this procedure.

REFERENCES

1. Saltzman CL, Salamon ML, Blanchard GM, et al. Epidemiology of ankle arthritis: report of a consecutive series of 639 patients from a tertiary orthopaedic center. Iowa Orthop J 2005;25:44–6.
2. Kluesner AJ, Wukich DK. Ankle arthrodiastasis. Clin Podiatr Med Surg 2009; 26(2):227–44.
3. Sagray BA, Levitt BA, Zgonis T. Ankle arthrodiastasis and interpositional ankle exostectomy. Clin Podiatr Med Surg 2012;29(4):501–7.
4. Stapleton JJ, Zgonis T. Supramalleolar osteotomy and ankle arthrodiastasis for juvenile posttraumatic ankle arthritis. Clin Podiatr Med Surg 2014;31(4): 597–601.

5. Kawoosa AA, Baba MA, Wani IH, et al. Ankle arthrodesis using the Ilizarov technique in difficult situations - a prospective study with mid-to long-term follow up. Ortop Traumatol Rehabil 2015;17(2):147–53.
6. Mongon ML, Garcia Costa KV, Bittar CK, et al. Tibiotalar arthrodesis in posttraumatic arthritis using the tension band technique. Foot Ankle Int 2013;34(6):851–5.
7. Gowda BN, Kumar JM. Outcome of ankle arthrodesis in posttraumatic arthritis. Indian J Orthop 2012;46(3):317–20.
8. Thiryayi WA, Naqui Z, Khan SA. Use of the Taylor spatial frame in compression arthrodesis of the ankle: a study of 10 cases. J Foot Ankle Surg 2010;49(2):182–7.
9. Zgonis T, Stapleton JJ, Roukis TS. Use of Taylor spatial frame for arthrodiastasis of the ankle joint. Tech Foot Ankle Surg 2007;6(3):201–7.
10. Nunley JA, Caputo AM, Easley ME, et al. Intermediate to long-term outcomes of the STAR Total Ankle Replacement: the patient perspective. J Bone Joint Surg Am 2012;94(1):43–8.
11. Saltzman CL, Kadoko RG, Suh JS. Treatment of isolated ankle osteoarthritis with arthrodesis or the total ankle replacement: a comparison of early outcomes. Clin Orthop Surg 2010;2(1):1–7.
12. Ellington JK, Gupta S, Myerson MS. Management of failures of total ankle replacement with the agility total ankle arthroplasty. J Bone Joint Surg Am 2013;95(23):2112–8.
13. Paley D, Lamm BM, Purohit RM, et al. Distraction arthroplasty of the ankle–how far can you stretch the indications? Foot Ankle Clin 2008;13(3):471–84.
14. Zgonis T, Stapleton JJ, Roukis TS. Use of circular external fixation for combined subtalar joint fusion and ankle distraction. Clin Podiatr Med Surg 2008;25(4):745–53.
15. Ramanujam CL, Sagray B, Zgonis T. Subtalar joint arthrodesis, ankle arthrodiastasis, and talar dome resurfacing with the use of a collagen-glycosaminoglycan monolayer. Clin Podiatr Med Surg 2010;27(2):327–33.
16. Fragomen AT, McCoy TH, Meyers KN, et al. Minimum distraction gap: how much ankle joint space is enough in ankle distraction arthroplasty? HSS J 2014;10(1):6–12.
17. Nguyen MP, Pedersen DR, Gao Y, et al. Intermediate-term follow-up after ankle distraction for treatment of end-stage osteoarthritis. J Bone Joint Surg Am 2015;97(7):590–6.
18. Castagnini F, Pellegrini C, Perazzo L, et al. Joint sparing treatments in early ankle osteoarthritis: current procedures and future perspectives. J Exp Orthop 2016;3(1):3.
19. Labovitz JM. The role of arthrodiastasis in salvaging arthritic ankles. Foot Ankle Spec 2010;3(4):201–4.
20. Rodriguez E, Hutchinson B, Clifford C, et al. Arthrodiastasis in the treatment of ankle arthritis: a case series. Foot Ankle Online J 2012;5(7):2.
21. Herrera-Pérez M, Pais-Brito JL, de Bergua-Domingo J, et al. Results of arthrodiastasis in postraumatic ankle osteoarthritis in a young population: prospective comparative study. Rev Esp Cir Ortop Traumatol 2013;57(6):409–16.
22. van Valburg AA, van Roermund PM, Marijnissen AC, et al. Joint distraction in treatment of osteoarthritis: a two-year follow-up of the ankle. Osteoarthritis Cartilage 1999;7(5):474–9.
23. Marijnissen AC, Van Roermund PM, Van Melkebeek J, et al. Clinical benefit of joint distraction in the treatment of severe osteoarthritis of the ankle: proof of concept in an open prospective study and in a randomized controlled study. Arthritis Rheum 2002;46(11):2893–902.

24. Ploegmakers JJ, van Roermund PM, van Melkebeek J, et al. Prolonged clinical benefit from joint distraction in the treatment of ankle osteoarthritis. Osteoarthritis Cartilage 2005;13(7):582–8.
25. Barg A, Amendola A, Beaman DN, et al. Ankle joint distraction arthroplasty: why and how. Foot Ankle Clin 2013;18(3):459–70.

Arthroscopic Treatment of Ankle Arthritis

Eric A. Barp, DPM[a],*, John G. Erickson, DPM[b], Jennifer L. Hall, DPM[c]

KEYWORDS

- Ankle arthroscopy • Ankle arthritis • Anterior ankle impingement
- Syndesmotic arthritis

KEY POINTS

- The goal of this article is to provide insight into evaluating and treating ankle arthritis.
- Types of pathologic ankle arthritis and their presentations are discussed.
- Ankle arthroscopy as a first-line treatment of ankle arthritis, its complications, and mid-term results are reported.

INTRODUCTION/HISTORY

Initial reports of arthroscopic procedures were described in 1918 by Kenji Takagi, who first placed an arthroscope in a knee joint. The ankle joint was largely considered unamenable to arthroscopic procedures until the 1970s, when Watanabe reported his experience with the procedure.[1] With recent technological advances in both instrumentation and optics, arthroscopy of the ankle has become commonplace with a multitude of abnormalities being able to be addressed. The goal of the current article is to provide a practical review of the indications, arthroscopic anatomy, abnormality-specific indications and considerations, technique, and complications for the arthroscopic treatment of ankle arthritis.

ANATOMY

The tibiotalar joint is a ginglymus joint that is largely responsible for sagittal plane motion in the foot. Normal range of motion (ROM) is typically noted to be 45° of plantar flexion and greater than 10° of dorsiflexion. The ankle mortise is formed by the tibial plafond and the medial and lateral malleoli. The tibial plafond is a concave structure that provides structural stability while allowing the motion necessary for ambulation. The

[a] Podiatry, The Iowa Clinic, 5950 University Avenue, West Des Moines, IA 50266, USA; [b] Podiatry, Boone County Hospital, 1015 Union Street, Boone, IA 50036, USA; [c] Podiatric Residency, UnityPoint Health-Des Moines, 1415 Woodland Avenue, Suite 100, Des Moines, IA 50309, USA
* Corresponding author.
E-mail address: ebarp@iowaclinic.com

Clin Podiatr Med Surg 34 (2017) 433–444
http://dx.doi.org/10.1016/j.cpm.2017.05.002
0891-8422/17/© 2017 Elsevier Inc. All rights reserved.

lateral aspect of the tibia includes the incisura fibularis, which is a concave structure that articulates with the fibula, comprising the lateral aspect of the mortise. The tibiofibular syndesmosis is structurally supported by the anterior inferior tibiofibular ligament, posterior inferior tibiofibular ligament, and the interosseous tibiofibular ligament. The ankle joint is then structurally supported by the deltoid ligament complex medially and the lateral collateral ligaments laterally. The deltoid ligament is divided into a deep and superficial layer. The deep deltoid ligament runs from the medial malleolus to the medial aspect of the talar body. The superficial deltoid ligament runs from the medial malleolus to the navicular and sustentaculum tali of the calcaneus, medial wall of the talus, and spring ligament. Lateral ankle ligaments consist of the anterior talofibular ligament, the calcaneofibular ligament, and the posterior talofibular ligament.

The anterior ankle anatomy is also relevant to review as the standard portals are placed to spare these vital structures. The most commonly damaged structure during arthroscopic surgery is the superficial peroneal nerve, which travels from the lateral leg to the dorsal foot and frequently can be damaged with the anterolateral portal. To a lesser degree, the saphenous nerve may be damaged because it runs just anterior to the medial malleolus with the saphenous vein. From medial to lateral, the tendinous structures that cross the anterior aspect of the ankle include the tibialis anterior, extensor hallucis longus, extensor digitorum longus, and peroneus tertius. The anterior tibial artery and deep peroneal nerve also course along the anterior ankle just deep to the extensor hallucis longus.

TECHNIQUE

Routine ankle arthroscopy is performed with the patient in a supine position with the foot elevated off of the bed. Positioning is accomplished with a leg holder or other positioning device. Portals are typically identified, marked, and placed in the anteromedial and anterolateral aspects of the ankle; however, the posterior medial and posterolateral approaches can also be used if abnormality indicates. The anterior medial portal is created 2 to 5 mm medial to the tibialis anterior tendon immediately inferior to the tibial plafond. The anterolateral portal is created just lateral to the peroneus tertius tendon at the level of the ankle joint (**Fig. 1**). The posterolateral incision is made just lateral to the Achilles tendon, 2 mm proximal to the tip of the fibula. The posteromedial portal is rarely indicated secondary to proximity of the posterior neurovascular bundle; if needed, it is placed just medial to the Achilles tendon at the same level as the posterolateral portal. A multitude of accessory portals have been described as well; however, each of these portals carries significant risk to adjacent structures and should be avoided.

Generally, the anterior medial portal is initially established with an 18-gauge needle, and the joint is insufflated with approximately 20 mL of lactated Ringers solution for distraction. Next, a small incision is made through the skin, and blunt dissection is performed to the joint capsule. A blunt obturator and cannula are used to gain access to the ankle joint without causing damage to the articular surfaces. The camera is inserted through this portal, and an initial examination of the ankle joint is performed. Typically, a 30° 2.7-mm arthroscope is used for this procedure; however, 4.0 mm and 70° scopes have uses as well. Depending on surgeon preference, a 2.7-mm or 3.5-mm shaver is used to debride the synovitis. The anterolateral portal is then created under direct visualization of the arthroscope, and using transillumination to ensure vital structures is avoided.

Once portals are established, a shaver is used to remove any hypertrophic synovium that allows for better visualization of the joint space. A blunt probe is frequently used to determine the viability of the articular cartilage, and any loose bodies are removed with a grasper. A 21-point inspection of the ankle joint (**Table 1**), as

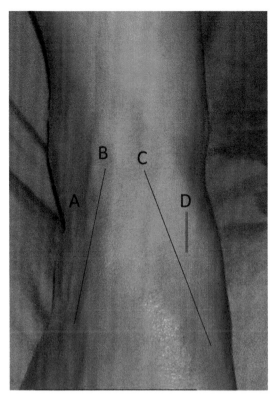

Fig. 1. (*A*) Lateral portal. (*B*) Peroneus tertius. (*C*) Anterior tibial tendon. (*D*) Medial portal.

described by Ferkel and colleagues,[2,3] should be performed, and any pathologic abnormalities should be addressed.

A thorough debridement and examination of the ankle joint can typically be performed without the necessity of distracting the ankle joint; however, there are times when

Table 1
Twenty-one-point arthroscopic examination of the ankle joint, as described by Ferkel

Anterior	Central	Posterior
Deltoid ligament	Medial tibia and talus	Posteromedial gutter
Medial gutter	Central tibia and talus	Posteromedial talus
Medial talus	Lateral tibiofibular and talofibular articulation	Posterocentral talus
Central talus	Posterior inferior tibiofibular ligament	Posterolateral talus
Lateral talus	Transverse ligament	Posterior talofibular articulation
Trifurcation of talus, tibia, fibula	Reflection of flexor hallucis longus	Posterolateral gutter
Lateral gutter		Posterior gutter
Anterior gutter		

Data from Ferkel RD. Arthroscopic surgery: the foot and ankle. Philadelphia: Lippincott-Raven; 1996. p. 85–103; and Ferkel RD, Heath DD, Guhl JF. Neurological complications of ankle arthroscopy. Arthroscopy 1996;12(2):200–8.

distraction is required. Several options have been described, including both noninvasive and invasive distraction techniques. Manual distraction is an option for most anterior abnormality, where an assistant provides distraction for a limited amount of time. More commonly, a commercially available noninvasive ankle strap is used. Yates and Grana[4] described a technique using a standard gauze roll wrapped around the surgeon's waist, allowing for controlled distraction periodically throughout the procedure. Invasive distraction has been described as well, consisting of a pin being placed into the tibia as well as the calcaneus. This distraction type is used only under rare circumstances where noninvasive distraction is not an option. Regardless of the distraction method selected, Dowdy and colleagues[5] recommended limiting distraction force to less than 30 pounds of pressure for less than an hour to reduce the risk of nerve damage.

GENERAL INDICATIONS

Ankle arthroscopy has many uses and indications among foot and ankle surgeons. The cause of ankle pain varies considerably from one patient to the next, making ankle arthroscopy a valid treatment option for many of these patients. General indications for arthroscopy include acute, recurring-acute, and chronic ankle pain with or without radiographic evidence of degeneration. Specific pathologic presentations and what to expect are discussed in detail later.

PATIENT EVALUATION

Clinical evaluation of the ankle joint begins with palpation of key anatomic structures in the ankle and surrounding joints. Arthritis may present with erythema and edema associated with the joint depending on severity of degeneration within the joint space. Three-view ankle radiographs are standard imaging; radiographs are not sensitive in the early stages of many arthritic disease processes.[6]

Diagnostic intra-articular local anesthetic injections can be used for diagnostic purposes. Injection of the anesthetic into the joint should alleviate pain for a few hours after injection. In patients whose pain dissipates, the pain is deemed to be related to the joint. If the pain remains, consider MRI for further evaluation. In addition, in severe cases or when other causes of pain are possible, MRI should be obtained.

Once the diagnosis of osteoarthritis is made, discussion of surgical versus conservative intervention should be done.

CONSERVATIVE THERAPY

Many patients presenting to the clinic with ankle arthritis have attempted at home therapies before their visit. Common reports include the following:

- Bracing (a variety of over-the-counter [OTC] options are available)
- Ice
- Anti-inflammatory/pain medications, such as naproxen, ibuprofen, aspirin, acetaminophen
- Topical creams (Aspercreme, Icy-Hot, newer OTC lidocaine patches)

As the provider, the above listed therapies are all acceptable treatments to consider and offer when initially working with the patient. For example, a figure-eight-style brace may provide enough support and restriction of motion to limit pain in low-activity patients, therefore avoiding surgery. Other options not available OTC include the following:

- Ankle functional orthosis
- Prescription topical creams

- Prescription oral anti-inflammatory medication
- Intra-articular steroid injections

Intra-articular steroid injections can be used to decrease inflammation and pain. Steroidal injections may be given 3 times per year. If injections are working well and the effective duration is approximately 4 months or more, this is an acceptable treatment. Once duration of effectiveness decreases to less than 3 months, surgical intervention may be discussed.

If conservative therapy fails to provide adequate relief, and determination to proceed with surgical intervention is made, arthroscopy may be considered.

SURGICAL INTERVENTION
Posttraumatic Arthritis

Posttraumatic ankle arthritis is accepted as the most common cause of ankle arthritis, with reports ranging from 70% to 80% of all ankle arthritis.[7] According to one retrospective study, 36% of patients with a history of open reduction and internal fixation of a traumatic ankle fracture had radiographic evidence of advanced arthritis, grade 3 or 4 on the Kellgren and Lawrence scale, at a median of 17.9 years after injury.[8] When these patients had 3 or more risk factors (Weber C fracture, increasing body mass index, age >30 at time of injury, associated medial malleolar fracture), the rate of ankle arthritis nearly doubled to 65%.[8] Posttraumatic ankle arthritis commonly presents as the following:

- Anterior ankle impingement (bony or soft tissue)
- Syndesmotic injury
- Osteochondral defects
- Loose bodies, associated with any of the above

Depending on injury and risk factors, these types of injury can be successfully treated with ankle arthroscopy, as discussed lataer.[9]

Anterior Ankle Impingement

Anterior ankle impingement can be debilitating depending on level of activity and can affect individuals of all body types, activity levels, and ages. A small bony or soft tissue impingement in an active individual can cause increased pain with activities using full ROM, such as running and jumping. Impingements of this type can lead to a significant lifestyle change in the active patient, and ankle arthroscopy may be of significant benefit to this population. Larger impingements can lead to a significant decrease in ROM, producing pain with simple activities such as walking, biking, or going down stairs. ROM may be increased with selective ankle arthroscopy and removal of bone and soft tissue impingements on the anterior tibia, fibula, and talus, leading to increased activity and patient satisfaction.

Soft tissue anterior ankle impingement (STAAI) is the inflammation or buildup of excess soft tissue within the ankle joint, including the following[10–12]:

- Capsular tissue (**Fig. 2**)
- Synovitic tissue (**Fig. 3**)
- Meniscoid lesion
- Bassett lesion, thickening of anterior inferior tibiofibular ligament at the anterior tibiotalar junction (**Fig. 4**)

When the ankle is taken through ROM, these tissues take up space in the anterior ankle, typically filled with synovial fluid, and stop the ankle before approaching full

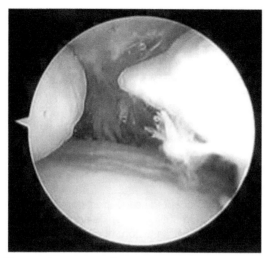

Fig. 2. Anterior ankle capsule overgrowth.

ROM.[13–15] The tissues are pinched between the bones and cause generalized discomfort, pressure, and pain within the ankle joint. Patients typically present with diffuse ankle pain and a catching feeling at end dorsiflexion. The degree of diminished end dorsiflexion is often variable depending on the degree of soft tissue impingement during each repetition. As the impingement progresses, synovitic material and capsular thickening continue to build, causing the pain and frequency of "catching"

A

B

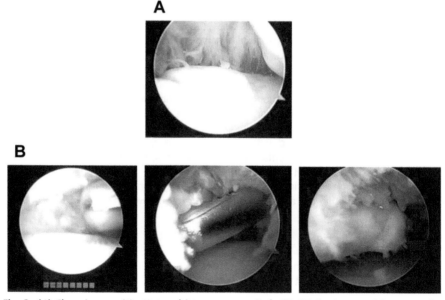

Fig. 3. (*A*) Chronic synovitis. Note white appearance of villi. (*B*) Acute synovitis entrapping on the anterior tibia. Note the red appearance of acute synovitis.

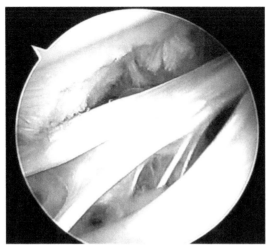

Fig. 4. Basset lesion.

to become more predictable and significant. Patients may have attempted bracing, ice, and anti-inflammatory medications at home with mild to moderate relief.

Examination of these patients will reveal decreased dorsiflexion with some repetitions and may not with others, because the soft tissues remain mobile.[15] There will often be pain with palpation along the anterior ankle joint space, where inflammation is present.[13,14] Patients typically do not recall a single traumatic episode.[15] Soft tissue impingements will not be visualized on plain films; however, plain films must be obtained to rule out potential bony abnormality. Further diagnostic imaging such as MRI can be used if necessary to more specifically determine cause of pain and rule out possible associated abnormalities, such as ligamentous or tendinous injury.

Bony anterior ankle impingement (BAAI) presents very similar to STAAI, with the exception that once large enough, the impingement causes a block at end dorsiflexion with each repetition at the same degree as can be measured with use of a goniometer. A palpable bony exostosis may be noted in more significant cases. The description by the patient may be one where the impingement progressively became worse over time and is now disrupting daily activities. There may have been one single traumatic episode recalled by the patient; however, this is not always the case as seen with repetitive microtrauma.[13,15] Global evaluation ensues, and plain films are obtained. Often, a bony exostosis will be visualized on lateral films at the anterior tibial lip and can be seen concomitantly with an opposite lesion at the talar neck, known as a kissing lesion (**Fig. 5**).[16] Less frequently seen on radiograph are anteromedial and anterolateral impingements, which can be associated with the talus, fibula, or tibia.[17] If radiographs are not sufficient for diagnosis, or if degeneration may be too complex for arthroscopy, proceeding to MRI or computed tomography is considered at this time to assist in proper surgical planning.

Whether the patient presents with BAAI or STAAI, workup should follow standard evaluations and imaging as necessary. Once a soft tissue or bony impingement is diagnosed, the surgeon may consider ankle arthroscopy as an appropriate means to remove the impingement, restoring a more anatomic ROM. Using standard anterior ankle arthroscopy portals, exploration of the entire joint is performed before beginning repair. If visualization is interrupted by significant arthritic changes, such as synovitic villi, a slight debridement using the arthroscopic shaver may take place to allow

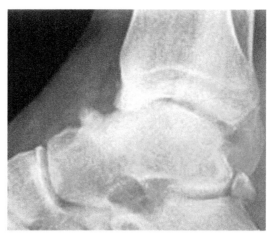

Fig. 5. Kissing lesion of the talus and tibia.

adequate visualization. Sufficient visualization of the joint surfaces is obtained for most problematic areas with inversion, eversion, dorsiflexion, and plantarflexion of the ankle used as tools for enhancing visualization. Once the ankle joint has been explored and no unexpected deformity is seen, debridement of soft tissue impingements can begin (**Fig. 6**). Meniscoid lesions, Bassett lesions, and acute and chronic synovitic villi (see **Figs. 3, 4**, and **6**) should be carefully debrided at this time using a soft tissue shaver or a variety of graspers. Once satisfied with soft tissue debridement, bone debridement ensues. It is possible to gain access to osteophytes and exostoses of the talar neck, anterior tibia, and medial and lateral gutters with careful manipulation of the arthroscope in combination with distraction and rotational maneuvers of the ankle. An arthroscopic bone reamer is used to remove bony overgrowth in problematic areas. Loose cartilage (**Fig. 7**) from partial or full-grade osteochondral defects (OCDs) can be removed at this time to prevent impingement in the future. As with any arthroscopic procedure, once the surgeon is satisfied with results, an additional scan of the joint should be performed to remove additional loose debris and to verify adequate ROM

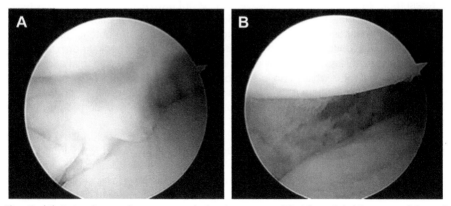

Fig. 6. (*A*) Lateral capsule overgrowth impingement. (*B*) After debridement of lateral capsule.

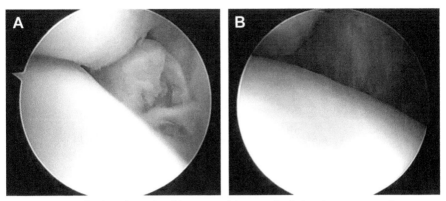

Fig. 7. (*A*) Loose body in lateral ankle gutter. (*B*) Loose body has been removed.

of the ankle joint. Instrumentation is removed from the ankle, and the ankle is taken through ROM a second time. Locking and decreased ROM before arthroscopy should now be resolved. It is important to advise the patient that the goal of the procedure is to increase ROM while decreasing swelling and pain. There may not be return to full ROM, or complete alleviation of pain with this procedure, although a significant increase in ROM should be obtained with adequate debridement.[9,17]

Successful talofibular impingement debridement alone via ankle arthroscopy has shown an average increase in ROM of 7.9°, measured intraoperatively, and American Orthopaedic Foot and Ankle Society score improved from 68.5 (range, 55–88) to 88.2 (range, 70–100).[17] A recent prospective 5-year study on arthroscopy for anterior impingement shows excellent results using the Functional Foot Index with a preoperative assessment mean of 20.5 and a postoperative mean of 2.7 at final follow-up.[9] Exostoses commonly recur within a 3- to 5-year follow-up; however, pain and functional levels typically do not reflect this recurrence.[9,13] Arthroscopy for anterior bony and soft tissue impingements has provided good to excellent short- to midterm results and currently is considered the gold standard of treatment of anterior ankle impingement.[9,13,17,18]

Syndesmotic Injury

Syndesmotic arthritis is commonly seen with the posttraumatic arthritic ankle. The latent syndesmotic injury is one where no syndesmotic widening is diagnosed on plain radiograph.[19] With this injury pattern, there remains minor laxity with ankle dorsiflexion for a period of time. When the syndesmosis does not self-stabilize and ≥2 mm diastasis remains, reactive synovitis builds into the syndesmosis (**Fig. 8**). As the synovitis continues to build, it eventually protrudes from into the joint becoming entrapped in the lateral gutter and lateral tibiotalar articulation, causing pain with ankle ROM.[20] Evaluation of the syndesmosis intraoperatively should be performed with any ankle arthroscopy. During the procedure, an assistant will lightly compress the fibula on the tibia, decreasing open space for the synovitis, which will then protrude into the joint and is easily debrided with a soft tissue shaver (see **Fig. 8**). The shaver can be inserted into the syndesmosis for additional debridement if needed (**Fig. 9**); this is typically done if the surgeon will be performing a syndesmotic stabilization during the case. Successful debridement results in decreased pain with ROM. Typically, if less than 4 mm, diastasis is visualized intraoperatively; debridement alone is sufficient to decrease pain and no syndesmotic stabilization is necessary.[20]

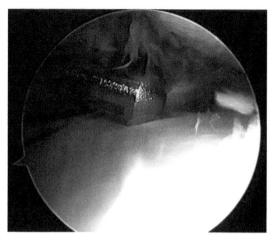

Fig. 8. Reactive synovitis protruding from the syndesmosis.

Osteochondral Defects

Frequently seen with posttraumatic arthritis, OCDs can prove to be very problematic for the patient. Significant pain and degeneration are often noted when an OCD is present. Often, a more rapid degeneration of the ankle joint is seen if there are loose bodies floating freely within the joint, causing further destruction and irritation of internal tissues. These free floating bodies continue the inflammatory cascade, causing continued pain. For some degree of OCD abnormality, ankle arthroscopy remains a viable, first-line therapy.

Primary Arthritis

Primary arthritis, also termed degenerative joint disease, or osteoarthritis, is described as generalized "wear and tear" affecting not just the hyaline cartilage of the joint but also eventually bony surfaces of the joint over time.[21] Typically, this type of arthritis begins to be bothersome and painful to patients when they enter their sixth and seventh decades of life and is rarely seen before the fourth decade.[7] Patients report no acute sports injury or other trauma in the past. Primary arthritis can be debilitating, like other forms of arthritis, especially in more active older adults. Prevalence of

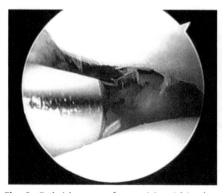
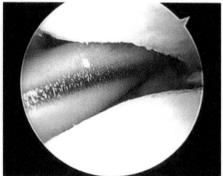

Fig. 9. Debridement of synovitis within the syndesmosis.

primary, or idiopathic, ankle arthritis is rare, accounting for only 7% of all types of ankle arthritis.[7,21] With such a low rate of occurrence, little literature is published on primary arthritis of the ankle and success rates with arthroscopy. Orthopedic literature on primary arthritis in the knee and hip suggests that arthroscopy is an acceptable treatment option. Using this information, and relatively good mid-term results of arthroscopic debridement of the posttraumatic ankle, it can be inferred that arthroscopy for primary ankle arthritis should be considered if fusion or replacement is not indicated at the time.

POSTOPERATIVE PERIOD

Postoperative protocols are dependent on the specific abnormality encountered and interventions performed. Most often, the postoperative protocol consists of non-weight-bearing in a CAM boot or posterior splint for 10 to 14 days, at which time the sutures are removed and ROM exercises are encouraged. If postoperative physical therapy is indicated, this typically is initiated 2 to 3 weeks postoperatively.

COMPLICATIONS

Although using the standard portals, complications of ankle arthroscopy are rare; however, they do still occur and range from less than 1% to 17%. A recent systematic review performed by Zwiers and colleagues[18] on arthroscopic treatment of anterior ankle impingement showed that the overall complication rate was 5.1% with 1.2% being considered major complications. Nerve injury is the most common complication, with the superficial peroneal nerve being the most commonly injured; however, the deep peroneal nerve, sural, saphenous, and tibial nerves can also be damaged. Neuroma formation can also be a significant cause of morbidity if a nerve is inadvertently transected. The risk of nerve injury is increased with prolonged distraction of the joint, full-thickness portal creation, repetitive replacement of instruments through portals, and utilization of the anterior central portal. Utilization of arthroscopic pumps increases the risk for extravasation of fluid into the soft tissue envelope. Unfortunately, the risk of iatrogenic cartilage damage due to instrumentation is likely underreported and difficult to assess. Other risk factors include infection, draining sinus tract with delayed healing of incision, tendon injury, and damage to the capsule and ligaments secondary to aggressive debridement. With meticulous dissection and rigorous surgical technique, most complications can be avoided.

SUMMARY

Arthroscopic treatment of ankle arthritis shows promising midterm results. All aspects of the pending arthroscopic surgery should be discussed with the patient, including complications, postoperative limitations, likelihood for future surgery as a fusion or replacement, and anticipated results. It is important to properly inform the patient that the desired postoperative outcome is allowing the patient to proceed with activity previously limited by pain and decreased ROM, but not to expect to be pain free or return to full ROM. Once carefully discussed, it is acceptable to proceed with arthroscopic ankle debridement, which is currently considered the gold standard first-line treatment of anterior ankle impingement.[18]

REFERENCES

1. Watanabe M. Selfoc arthroscopy (Watanabe no 24 arthroscopes) monograph. Tokyo: Teishin Hospital; 1972.

2. Ferkel RD. Arthroscopic surgery: the foot and ankle. Philadelphia: Lippincott-Raven; 1996. p. 85–103.
3. Ferkel RD, Heath DD, Guhl JF. Neurological complications of ankle arthroscopy. Arthroscopy 1996;12(2):200–8.
4. Yates CK, Grana WA. A simple distraction technique for ankle arthroscopy. Arthroscopy 1988;4:103–5.
5. Dowdy PA, Watson BV, Amendola A, et al. Noninvasive ankle distraction: relationship between force, magnitude of distraction and nerve conduction abnormalities. Arthroscopy 1996;12:64–9.
6. Hunter DJ, Mcdougall JJ, Keefe FJ. The symptoms of osteoarthritis and the genesis of pain. Med Clin North Am 2009;93(1):83–100, xi.
7. Saltzman CL, Salamon ML, Blanchard GM, et al. Epidemiology of ankle arthritis: report of a consecutive series of 639 patients from a tertiary orthopaedic center. Iowa Orthop J 2005;25:44–6.
8. Lübbeke A, Salvo D, Stern R, et al. Risk factors for post-traumatic osteoarthritis of the ankle: an eighteen year follow-up study. Int Orthop 2012;36(7):1403–10.
9. Walsh SJ, Twaddle BC, Rosenfeldt MP, et al. Arthroscopic treatment of anterior ankle impingement: a prospective study of 46 patients with 5-year follow-up. Am J Sports Med 2014;42(11):2722–6.
10. Bassett FH III, Gates HS III, Billys JB, et al. Talar impingement by the anteroinferior tibiofibular ligament. A cause of chronic pain in the ankle after inversion sprain. J Bone Joint Surg Am 1990;72:55–9.
11. Thein R, Eichenblat M. Arthroscopic treatment of sports related synovitis of the ankle. Am J Sports Med 1992;20:496–8.
12. Meislin RJ, Rose DJ, Parisien JS, et al. Arthroscopic treatment of synovial impingement of the ankle. Am J Sports Med 1993;21:186–9.
13. Tol JL, van Dijk CN. Anterior ankle impingement. Foot Ankle Clin 2006;11: 297–310, vi.
14. Kim SH, Ha KI. Arthroscopic treatment for impingement of the anterolateral soft tissues of the ankle. J Bone Joint Surg Br 2000;82(7):1019–21.
15. Baums MH, Kahl E, Schultz W, et al. Clinical outcome of the arthroscopic management of sports-related "anterior ankle pain": a prospective study. Knee Surg Sports Traumatol Arthrosc 2006;14(5):482–6.
16. Kitaoka HB. Master techniques in orthopaedic surgery: the foot and ankle. Philadelphia: Lippincott Williams & Wilkins; 2013. p. 515.
17. Ahn JY, Choi HJ, Lee WC. Talofibular bony impingement in the ankle. Foot Ankle Int 2015;36(10):1150–5.
18. Zwiers R, Wiegerinck JI, Murawski CD, et al. Arthroscopic treatment for anterior ankle impingement: a systematic review of the current literature. Arthroscopy 2015;31(8):1585–96.
19. Edwards GS, Delee JC. Ankle diastasis without fracture. Foot Ankle 1984;4(6): 305–12.
20. Ryan PM, Rodriguez RM. Outcomes and return to activity after operative repair of chronic latent syndesmotic instability. Foot Ankle Int 2016;37(2):192–7.
21. Felson DT. An update on the pathogenesis and epidemiology of osteoarthritis. Radiol Clin North Am 2004;42(1):1–9, v.

Supramalleolar Osteotomies

Varun Chopra, DPM, Paul Stone, DPM*, Alan Ng, DPM

KEYWORDS

- Supramalleolar osteotomy • Ankle arthritis • Asymmetric ankle arthritis
- Varus ankle or valgus ankle • Ankle realignment

KEY POINTS

- A supramalleolar osteotomy is a joint-sparing osteotomy that can correct deformities in all planes at the distal tibia.
- Supramalleolar osteotomies have been found to provide substantial pain relief and functional improvement.
- With proper patient selection and preoperative planning, the supramalleolar osteotomy can effectively redistribute the forces placed on the ankle with the goal of limiting progression of degenerative changes.

INTRODUCTION

Distal tibial malalignment can result from posttraumatic malunion, physeal disturbances, congenital or metabolic diseases, and degenerative arthritis. The load-bearing area of the ankle is smaller than that of the knee, which leads to an increase in load per unit area. Kimizuka and colleagues[1] reported that when a force of 500 N was applied, the area of contact in the ankle was 350 mm^2 compared with 1100 mm^2 in the hip and 1120 mm^2 in the knee. For this reason, osteoarthritis (OA) readily develops once a structural abnormality is present. Approximately 15% of the world's adult population is affected by joint pain resulting from OA and approximately 1% have OA of the ankle.[2] Around 80% of the cases of arthritis of the ankle are posttraumatic and tends to effect more young people compared with those with hip and knee arthritis.[3]

Procedures treating ankle arthritis can be divided into 2 categories: joint-preserving and joint-sacrificing procedures. Joint-preserving procedures include ankle arthroscopy/arthrotomy with joint debridement,[4] distraction arthroplasty,[5] partial or total osteochondral resurfacing procedures,[6] and alignment corrective osteotomies.[7]

Disclosure Statement: None.
PMSR/RRA, Highlands/Presbyterian St. Luke's Podiatric Surgical Residency Program, 1719 East 19th Avenue, Denver, CO 80218, USA
* Corresponding author.
E-mail address: pstonehighlandspslresidency@comcast.net

Joint-sacrificing procedures include ankle arthrodesis[8] and total ankle replacement.[9,10] Malalignment of the ankle leads to an altered load distribution across the joint, interfering with normal cartilage metabolism leading to early ankle joint arthritis that usually presents asymmetrically.[11] For patients where a substantial part of the joint is still salvageable, ankle fusion or joint replacement is not always the best option. For this patient population, realignment osteotomy of the distal tibia is a valuable procedure.

A supramalleolar osteotomy is a joint-sparing osteotomy that can correct deformities in all planes at the distal tibia. The goals of supramalleolar osteotomy are to realign the ankle and foot to the leg to transfer the ankle joint under the weightbearing axis and to normalize the direction of the force vector of the triceps surae. Restoring the axial alignment allows for redistribution of loads to an area where the articular cartilage is less affected to slow down further articular degeneration. Several studies have found the successes of the osteotomy in improving function and relieving pain.

HISTORY OF SUPRAMALLEOLAR OSTEOTOMY

In 1936, Speed and Boyd, orthopedic surgeons who presented their treatment algorithm for posttraumatic deformities above the ankle joint.[12] They published a clinical study that included 50 realignment surgeries in patients with posttraumatic deformities. They determined 3 crucial aims of supramalleolar realignment surgical procedures[1]: restoration of appropriate weight-bearing alignment of the leg,[2] restoration of the appropriate alignment of articulating surfaces of the tibiotalar joint, and[3] restoration of physiologic and pain-free range of motion of the tibiotalar joint.

One of the first publications to report outcomes of a supramalleolar osteotomy came from Saint Petersburg in 1966 by Dzakhov and Kurochkin, titled "Supramalleolar osteotomies in children and adolescents."[13] The authors presented their results in 59 patients who underwent supramalleolar realignment osteotomy between 1936 and 1964. Another early article on supramalleolar osteotomy was published by Barskii and Semenov from Kujbyshev, Russia in 1979. In their publication, "Methods of the supramalleolar osteotomy in ununited fractures of the malleoli," the authors described their surgical technique and preoperative planning for a medial closing-wedge supramalleolar osteotomy.[14]

Most review articles detail a historical perspective on supramalleolar osteotomy; a study by Takakura and colleagues[15] in 1995 is noted as the first to report outcomes systematically in patients who underwent supramalleolar osteotomy. They are considered the pioneers of this field and their work substantially influenced the work of many foot and ankle surgeons. Since Takakura's report, an increasing number of clinical studies of patients who have undergone supramalleolar osteotomies have been published. Overall studies consistently show good short-term and midterm results for pain relief, functional improvement, and return to sports and recreation activities.

BIOMECHANICS

There is no consensus in the literature regarding the degree of distal tibial malalignment and the potential for development of arthritis and symptoms. Tarr and colleagues[16] established that distal deformities with an angulation of 15° showed up to a 42% reduction in contact area. However, another study by Kristensen and colleagues,[17] who looked at patients with low tibia fractures with greater than 10° angular malunion, found that many of the patients were asymptomatic and none of the patients had limitations of ankle motion. Their patients also had no radiographic signs of ankle arthrosis 20 years after injury.

Many studies have shown that the ability of subtalar joint to compensate deformity above the ankle as a main factor for the foot and ankle to be able to tolerate distal tibial deformity. The available amount of motion in the subtalar joint can vary considerably between patients.[18,19] Paley[20] believes 30° of angle valgus and 15° of ankle varus can be compensated with a normal functioning subtalar joint. Distal tibial valgus is typically better compensated than distal tibial varus owing to there being twice as much available inversion in the subtalar joint than eversion.

INDICATIONS AND CONTRAINDICATIONS

Distal tibial malalignment is often the result of a previous physeal disturbance from a trauma in childhood, a pilon fracture, a distal tibial shaft fracture leading to degenerative arthritis, or a congenital or metabolic disturbance. A majority of patients with ankle OA have a posttraumatic etiology.[21] Posttraumatic ankle arthritis consists of a progressive alteration of the hyaline cartilage, sclerosis of the subchondral bone, and formation of osteophytes and loose bodies.[22] Malalignment can occur in the coronal plane (varus and valgus) as well as the sagittal plane (flexion and extension). Malalignment changes the mechanical axis and altering load distribution to cause asymmetric overload of the articular surface. Additionally, trauma often leads to direct cartilage shear or impaction that also may lead to ankle arthritis.[23]

Indications

- Aysmmetric ankle OA with angular deformity
- Physeal growth arrest
- Tibial fracture malunion
- Ankle arthrodesis malunion
- Rheumatoid ankle
- Paralytic deformities
- Hemophilic arthropathy
- Total ankle arthroplasty realignment

Contraindications

Proper patient selection is the key to the success of a supramalleolar osteotomy. There are relative and absolute contraindications for supramalleolar osteotomy, which include the following.

Absolute contraindications

- End-stage degenerative with less than 50% of tibiotalar joint surface preserved
- Unmanageable hindfoot instability
- Acute or chronic infections
- Severe vascular or neurologic deficiency
- Neuropathic disorders

Relative contraindications

- Advanced age
- Impaired bone quality of the distal tibia and/or talus
- Tobacco use owing to an expected higher rate of osseous nonunion

In patients with contraindications to joint-preserving osteotomies, arthrodesis of the ankle joint or total ankle arthroplasty are viable alternative treatment options.

CLINICAL PRESENTATION

Clinical evaluation should include a complete history, with particular note of prior trauma, physical testing, and diagnostic evaluation. The most important aspect of pre-operative planning is assessment of the origin of deformity and understanding of the deforming forces. It is important to test hindfoot stability during the routine physical examination because, as noted, having adequate subtalar joint range of motion and flexibility is critical. There is also a risk of unmasking adaptive deformity in the subtalar joint when realigning the ankle joint, which is why a thorough examination is needed.[24] Function of the peroneal tendons in the varus ankle and the posterior tibial tendon in the valgus ankle also needs to be assessed. Other components of the physical examination should include assessment of the range of motion of the ankle joint, as well as evaluation of forefoot deformities, such as a plantarflexed first ray, forefoot supination, and toe deformities.

RADIOGRAPHIC EVALUATION

Radiographs should include weightbearing assessment of the foot and ankle, hindfoot alignment, and long leg calcaneal axial views. The contralateral extremity should also be evaluated to understand fully the location and degree of deformity. Other imaging modalities useful in evaluation and surgical planning include computed tomography (CT) scans, MRI, and single-photon emission CT. CT scanning is helpful in accurately measuring the length of the tibia and fibula as well as identifying any malrotation. MRI is used to analyze the soft tissue and articular cartilage. Single-photon emission to-mography CT scans can give the surgeon an idea of areas with increased tibiotalar joint pressures.

The anteroposterior (AP) and lateral views help to determine the type and degree of deformity in all planes. Using concepts of vector trigonometry described by Paley,[25] supramalleolar osteotomy can be planned and executed with predictable re-sults by obtaining accurate radiographic angles. The center of the ankle joint and the middiaphyseal line extended to the joint are important parameters to be familiar with. In a rectus ankle, the middiaphyseal line should pass through the center of the talus on the AP view and the lateral talar process on the lateral view. These landmarks form joint orientation angles; the anterior distal tibial angle and the lateral distal tibial angle.

The mechanical (anatomic) axis of the distal tibia is the extension of the mechanical axis of the lower extremity. The mechanical axis distally extends through the center of the ankle joint. The angle formed by the tibial plafond on the AP view and the mechanical axis of the tibia is called the distal tibial ankle surface angle and is typically 93°. On the lateral radiograph, this angle is referred to as the tibial lateral surface angle, nor-mally averaging 80° (**Fig. 1**). When performing a distal tibial osteotomy, the goal is to restore the tibial ankle surface angle and tibial lateral surface angle back to within normal values, similar to the contralateral limb.

Frontal plane radiographs are used to evaluate the calcaneus to tibial relation-ship. On a weightbearing long leg calcaneal axial and hindfoot alignment radio-graph, the tibial middiaphyseal line should parallel the calcaneal bisection line. On the hindfoot alignment view, the normal heel bisection is 5 to 10 mm lateral to the tibial middiaphyseal line. A subtalar joint deformity is seen on the long leg calca-neal axial view and an osseous calcaneal tuber deformity is visualized on the hind-foot alignment view. Therefore, both frontal plane radiographs are critical to appropriately assess the preoperative alignment/relationship between the talus, tibia, and calcaneus.

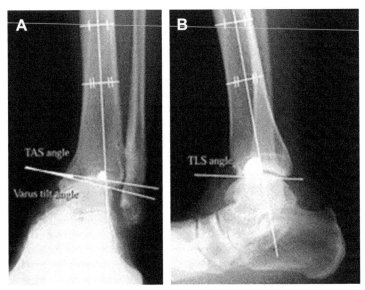

Fig. 1. Radiographic measurement. TAS, tibial anterior surface angle; TLS, tibial lateral surface angle.

Other radiographic findings on the AP and lateral radiographs that are useful in preoperative planning are the evaluation of the articular surface, loose joint bodies, osteophytes, and bony defects. If the possibility of a nonunion is present from a prior injury or surgery, a preoperative CT scan can be useful.

CENTER OF ROTATION AND ANGULATION ANALYSIS

Every deformity has an apex of the deformity. This apex is referred to as the center of rotation and angulation (CORA). The CORA is used as a reference point for osteotomy planning and the location of the CORA is determined by the intersection of 2 lines that represent the mechanical axes of the proximal and distal segments. In cases with isolated angular deformity, the CORA is at the apex of the deformity. When a translation deformity is also present, the CORA is located above the level of the deformity. Often, the level of the CORA will be different on the AP and lateral films, which results in translation in a different plane from the plane of the angulation deformity.

Paley[25] described 3 osteotomy rules that should be used to predict the level of osteotomy to give you expected results based on the location of the osteotomy relative to the CORA. Violation of these rules may result in a secondary iatrogenic deformity and in general the supramalleolar osteotomy should be placed as at or close to CORA as possible.

Osteotomies rules include the following.

Rule 1: When the osteotomy and axis of correction of angulation pass through the CORA, pure angulation correction occurs without translation.

Rule 2: When the axis of correction of angulation is through the CORA but the osteotomy is at a different level, the deformity realigns by angulation and translation at the osteotomy site.

Rule 3: When the osteotomy and axis of correction of angulation are at a level away from the CORA, a translation deformity results.

SURGICAL PLANNING

Surgical planning requires an understanding of normal lower limb alignment and joint orientation. First, planning consists of defining the anatomic axis of the tibia on the AP and lateral views. Next, it is necessary to determine the lateral distal tibial angle and anterior distal tibial angle, which, when extended proximally, define the CORA. Finally, evaluation of the hindfoot alignment with respect to the tibial axis and ankle joint is needed. Once the surgeon has defined the deformity, level of the CORA, and hindfoot position, clinical examination should determine rotation, soft tissue contracture, and ligament instability. With this complete information, proper deformity correction with the appropriate procedures can be performed (see **Fig. 1**; **Fig. 2**).

CALCULATING THE DEGREE OF CORRECTION

Preoperative planning also necessitates calculation of wedge resection or the quantity of bone graft needed to achieve the desired degree of correction. To calculate the degree of correction needed an equation that results in a 1:1 ratio of degrees correct to millimeters of wedge resection or grafting is used. The equation consists of calculating the height of the wedge to be resected or grafted, the magnitude of deformity, and the width of the tibia at the level of the osteotomy.[26,27]

$H\ 5\ tan\ a1\ W$

Where H is the height of the wedge to be resected or grafted; $a1$ is the magnitude of deformity plus the degrees of overcorrection; and W is the width of the tibia at the level of the osteotomy.

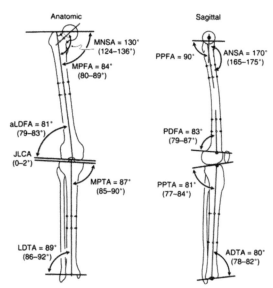

Fig. 2. Normal joint orientation angles and anatomic axes in the frontal and sagittal planes. ADTA, anterior distal tibial angle; aLDFA, anatomic lateral distal femoral angle; ANSA, anterior neck shaft angle; JLCA, joint line convergence angle; LDTA, lateral distal tibial angle; mLDFA, mechanical lateral distal femoral angle; MNSA, medial neck shaft angle; MPFA, medial proximal femoral angle; MPTA, medial proximal tibial angle; PDFA, posterior distal femoral angle; PPFA, posterior proximal femoral angle; PPTA, posterior proximal tibial angle.

OSTEOTOMY SELECTION

It is important to know the advantages and disadvantages of the different osteotomies available. There are 3 main options to correct varus or valgus deformity of the ankle. Options include open or closing wedge osteotomies or focal dome osteotomy. Typically, lateral osteotomies are avoided owing to it being relatively difficult to perform because of the close proximity of the fibula. However, most believe that, when greater than 10° of correction is needed, a lateral wedge osteotomy is typically preferred. Mulhern and colleagues[28] reported advantages and disadvantages of common supramalleolar osteotomies, results are in **Table 1**. Disadvantages of lateral closing wedge osteotomies not listed in Mulhern's table include more extensive soft tissue dissection, possible weakening of the peroneals, and a possible leg shortening in large corrections.[34]

SURGICAL TECHNIQUE

In general, supramalleolar osteotomies are performed through a medial, anterior, or lateral approach. It is important to evaluate the local soft tissue conditions and the presence of previous incisions or wounds. General anesthesia is often used in conjunction with regional or spinal anesthetics. In general, it is important to avoid stripping excessive amounts of the periosteal layer to prevent devascularization of the osteotomy site. The transverse design and metaphyseal location of the osteotomy is helpful, because it is inherently stable in an area of good blood supply for rapid healing.

It remains controversial as to which type of osteotomy should be performed in patients with supramalleolar varus deformity: lateral closing wedge osteotomy or medial opening wedge osteotomy. The decision is mainly based on the surgeon's preference. The medial approach is easier to perform; however, in a patient with preoperative varus deformity of more than 10°, an appropriate correction often cannot be achieved with a tibial osteotomy alone because the fibula may restrict the degree of supramalleolar correction.

OPENING AND CLOSING WEDGE OSTEOTOMY

In general, for correction of varus or valgus deformity use a half pin percutaneously placed as near to the CORA as possible in the distal metaphyseal region of the tibia to serve as the center of rotation for the osteotomy. When the CORA falls at the ankle joint, the pin cannot be placed in the joint but can be placed just proximal, which will cause some translation. The osteotomy is performed in metaphyseal bone and the guide hole that is used is the one that will provide the ability for the osteotomy to exit both the medial and lateral cortexes of the tibia. Multiple holes are made along the planned osteotomy line, and then completed using an osteotome or saw blade to connect the holes.

The technique of a lateral closed wedged osteotomy includes a 10- to 12-cm longitudinal incision along the anterior margin of the distal fibula. Both the fibula and the tibia are exposed laterally as well as the anterior syndesmosis distally. In most cases of a varus deformity, the fibula is shortened to preserve the congruency in the ankle joint. This is done with a bone block removal or Z-shaped osteotomy. K-wires are then drilled through the tibia, converging at the medial cortex, and the osteotomy is performed and secured with a plate. Finally, the fibula is secured with screws or a one-third tubular plate.

A medial approach is used for medial opening osteotomies. The technique involves a midline incision along the distal medial metaphysis posterior to the great saphenous vein and saphenous nerve. The tibia is exposed, ensuring not to strip the periosteum. Using fluoroscopy, a guidewire is placed from medial to lateral in the plane of the osteotomy determined by the preoperative plan. The osteotomy is then completed

Table 1
Disadvantages and advantages of supramalleolar osteotomies

Approach	Correction	Advantages	Disadvantages	Considerations
Medial opening wedge	Varus to valgus (<10° varus)	• Allows multiplane correction with saw blade angulation[29,30] • Preserves limb length[27,31]	• Requires bone grafting; increased risk of nonunion[31] • Increased risk of neurovascular compromise[31]	• Consider concomitant tarsal tunnel release[20,32] • Translation is medial[29]
Medial closing wedge	Valgus to varus (any degree deformity)	• Allows multiplane correction with saw blade angulation[29] • Decreased risk of neurovascular compromise[31] • Decreased risk of nonunion because no bone graft is used[33]	• Results in shortening of limb length[31]	• Translation is lateral[20]
Lateral closing wedge	Varus to valgus (>10° varus)	• Allows multiplane correction with saw blade angulation[29] • Decreased risk of nonunion because no bone graft is used[33]	• Single-plane correction[29]	• Translation is medial[20]
Focal dome	Valgus to varus or varus to valgus	• Ideal for frontal/sagittal plane deformity with center of rotation and angulation at level of the ankle joint or in the talus[29] • Preserves limb length[32] • No thermal necrosis[32] • Minimal periosteal dissection[32] • Excellent bone to bone contact[32]		• Should be performed in metaphyseal bone[20]

Adapted from Mulhern J, Protzman N, Brigido SA, et al. Supramalleolar osteotomy: indications and surgical techniques. Clin Podiatr Med Surg 2015;32(3):453; with permission.

using a wide saw blade and the correction is made, typically preserving the lateral cortex to enhance the intrinsic stability. The tibial osteotomy is then gently distracted using a lamina spreader and the space is filled with an appropriately sized bone graft. In cases of sagittal plane deformity, an anterior or posterior medial wedge can be performed in a biplanar fashion. Rigid plate fixation with locking screws is recommended to secure the osteotomy. After the supramalleolar correction, the alignment of the heel is reassessed clinically. The aim is to achieve a heel with 1° to 5° valgus.

The anterior approach is used in patients with altered medial/lateral soft tissue quality or sagittal plane deformity. A longitudinal incision is made between the anterior tibial tendon and the extensor hallucis longus tendon starting from 10 cm proximal to the joint, about midway between the malleoli. Care must be taken to avoid the neurovascular bundle that lies lateral to the incision. The anterior surface of the tibia is then exposed and the osteotomy is carried out.

FOCAL DOME OSTEOTOMY

A focal dome osteotomy is typically used for frontal or sagittal plane correction at or near the ankle joint. It is placed in the metaphyseal bone and often needs additional fibular shortening. It can be performed open or percutaneously through multiple stab incisions. For open correction, a straight anterior incision is used between the extensor halluces longus and extensor digitorum longus tendons. An axis pin is placed in the distal tibial metaphysis ideally at the CORA to avoid producing a secondary deformity. A Rancho cube is used over the pin to allow circular rotation outlining the arc of the osteotomy. The holes in the cube are drilled and connected with an osteotome. An osteotomy of the fibula is then performed to allow mobilization of the distal fragment. Most often, a concomitant fibular osteotomy is also required. This can be achieved in an oblique fashion in the same plane as the correction or shortening can be performed if needed, using a cylindrical shortening osteotomy.

There are several options for fixation. Percutaneous cannulated or solid core screws or locking plate for a more rigid construct. Compression through the osteotomy with a tensioning deice can promote faster biological healing.

CONCOMITANT PROCEDURES

A neutral alignment within the ankle joint is crucial for positive results. When a residual talar varus or valgus tilt is observed a fibular osteotomy or plafondplasty may be needed. Occasionally, additional lateralizing or medializing calcaneal osteotomies may be required to achieve full realignment. Soft tissue contractures may inhibit correction, so release or reconstruction of the medial and lateral ligaments may be necessary. Posttraumatic medial soft tissue tightness may also cause tension on the neurovascular structures, and in these cases a prophylactic tarsal tunnel release is an option to consider (**Table 2**).

CASE STUDIES
Case Study 1

A 71-year-old woman presents with severe arthrosis with a varus malunion of the left ankle secondary to trauma. Her initial injury occurred when a Murphy bed fell

Table 2
Common concomitant procedures

Malalignment	Soft Tissue Procedures	Bony Procedures
Varus	Deltoid release, repair/ reconstruction of lateral ankle ligaments	Lateralizing calcaneal osteotomy, plafondplasty, fibular valgus osteotomy
Valgus	Repair/reconstruction of deltoid, spring ligament, and posterior tibial tendon; release of lateral ligaments	Medializing calcaneal osteotomy, medial malleolus varus osteotomy

on the left leg, leading to a comminuted fracture of the fibula. Since the injury, the patient has complained of severe deformity and instability. She states she has tried ankle braces but continues to have pain. Physical examination showed left leg in significant varus and a resting calcaneal stance position of 7° of valgus. Lateral instability noted as well as limited ankle joint range of motion. Radiographs revealed 15° of varus deformity as well as medial shoulder and gutter arthrosis at the ankle. Three surgical options were discussed with the patient, including ankle arthrodesis, ankle joint replacement arthroplasty, and supramalleolar osteotomy for decompression of the joint and repair of varus malposition. The patient elected for the ankle joint salvage procedure. The procedure performed included an opening wedge distal tibial osteotomy using a tantalum bone wedge and malleolar plate for fixation. The patient also had a prophylactic tarsal tunnel release and an Evans lateral ankle stabilization procedure. Postoperatively, the patient was kept non–weight bearing for 8 weeks and transitioned to partial weight bearing in a controlled ankle motion boot for an additional 2 weeks. At 10 weeks postoperative, the patient was allowed to bear weight as tolerated. At 6 months postoperative, the patient's pain and swelling had minimized and CT scans revealed consolidation of tantalum bone wedge (**Fig. 3**).

Case Study 2

A 68-year-old woman with a past medical history of rheumatoid arthritis on methotrexate presented to the clinic 1 year status post right ankle fracture from outside clinic. Patient suffered distal metaphyseal fracture of the tibia and Wb C fibular fracture with syndesmotic displacement. Patient is neurovascularly intact. The right ankle was edematous and there was a valgus malposition of the ankle and subtalar joint. The patient had normal ankle joint range of motion and limited subtalar joint range of motion. Preoperative radiographs of the right foot and ankle reveal severe valgus malposition of the ankle; however, the ankle joint is relatively intact (**Fig. 4**). The subtalar joint has severe arthrosis noted. The surgical plan was to perform a subtalar joint arthrodesis and repair of the malposition fracture using lateral approach supramalleolar and fibular osteotomy. By 6 months postoperative, the patient had boney union of osteotomy sites; however, the patient had a nonhealing wound and infection of the lateral incision

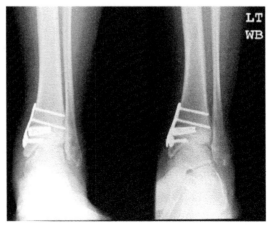

Fig. 3. Anteroposterior and MO views of left ankle at 6 months postoperative. Consolidation of medial opening wedge using tantalum bone wedge and malleolar plate.

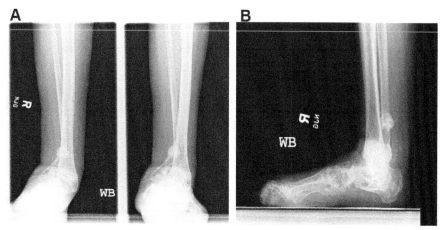

Fig. 4. *(A, B)* Preoperative radiographs of the right ankle. Severely valgus malposition of the right ankle. Ankle joint preserved. Subtalar joint severely arthritic.

(**Fig. 5**). The patient required hardware removal, wound care, and a free flap that healed uneventfully.

LITERATURE REVIEW

Overall, supramalleolar osteotomies have been found to provide substantial pain relief and functional improvement. Published results of supramalleolar osteotomies for both

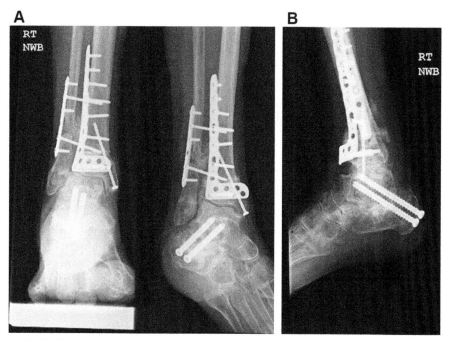

Fig. 5. *(A, B)* Radiographs of the of supramalleolar osteotomy at 6 months postoperatively using the lateral approach with fibular osteotomy and subtalar joint arthrodesis.

Table 3
Current literature on supramalleolar osteotomies

Study	Patients/Methods	Results	Complications
Pagenstert et al,[35] 2007	• Described treatment algorithm in 35 patients with varus or valgus OA	• Mean follow-up of 5 y AOFAS hindfoot scale significantly improved from 38.5 ± 17.2 preoperatively to 85.4 ± 12.4 postoperatively	• Revision surgery was necessary in 10 ankles
Hintermann et al,[36] 2008	• Described their treatment algorithm in 74 patients who underwent supramalleolar osteotomies	• Mean follow-up of 4.1 y • AOFAS hindfoot score significantly improved from 29 preoperatively to 84 postoperatively	• <5% required arthrodesis or total ankle replacement
Gessmann et al,[37] 2009	• Used the Taylor spatial frame external fixator for correction of complex supramalleolar deformities in 9 patients • The mean preoperative angular deformity was 30°	• Mean follow-up of 1.9 y • Anatomic restoration of the hindfoot alignment was achieved in all patients	• There were 2 pin-tract infections, 1 prolongated callus formation, and 1 insufficient callus formation
Hintermann et al,[38] 2011	• Studied patients with malunited pronation–external rotation fractures of the ankle • 45 patients were treated with a medial closing-wedge osteotomy • 3 patients treated with a lateral opening-wedge osteotomy	• Mean follow-up of 7.1 y • Good or excellent results were obtained in 42 patients (87.5%) with the benefit being maintained over time • Majority of patients could return to their former professional and sports activities	• 3 patients had considerable degenerative changes of the ankle • One patient required total ankle replacement
Knupp et al,[39] 2011	• Presented detailed classification/treatment algorithm of supramalleolar deformities based on clinical findings • 92 patients with asymmetric ankle OA were included in the study	• Mean follow-up 3.6 y • All osteotomies healed within 12 wk • No cases of nonunion • AOFAS hindfoot score and VAS score improved significantly • Patients with valgus ankles with fibular malalignment and varus ankles with concomitant ankle joint instability tended to have worse outcomes	• Ten ankles had to be converted to total ankle replacement or ankle arthrodesis

Study			
Lee et al,[40] 2011	• Reported results in 16 ankles treated with supramalleolar osteotomy combined with fibula osteotomy secondary to moderate medial ankle arthritis	• Mean follow-up of 2.3 y • The mean AOFAS score, mean Takakura stage, and mean values of all radiographic parameters were improved significantly after surgery	• Patients with lateral subfibular pain had a lower mean AOFAS score
Knupp et al,[41] 2012	• Reported results of realignment surgery in patients with overcorrected clubfoot deformity	• Mean follow-up of 4.2 y • All osteotomies healed within 8 wk • All patients experienced significant pain relief and functional improvement	• None
Barg et al,[42] 2013	• Reported on 42 patients with asymmetric posttraumatic ankle OA • 26 had valgus deformity treated with medial closing-wedge osteotomy • Patients with varus deformity were treated by medial opening-wedge[10] or lateral closing-wedge[4]	• All supramalleolar osteotomies healed within 4 mo	• None
Colin et al,[43] 2014	• Reported results of 83 patients with post-traumatic asymmetric early arthritis of the ankle • Looked for clinical "sidewalk sign"; considered positive if pain improved when patient walked on a surface slope that was tilted in opposite direction of deformity	• Mean follow-up of 3.5 y • AOFAS score significantly improved by 15 points in patients with a varus deformity and 13 points in patients with a valgus deformity • A positive sidewalk sign was correlated with a good outcome and had a positive predictive value	• 7 patients had complications, which included impingement, scar dehiscence, overcorrection, arthritis, nonunion, septic nonunion, and sepsis

Abbreviations: AOFAS, American Orthopaedic Foot and Ankle Society; OA, osteoarthritis; VAS, visual analog scale.

varus and valgus deformity have been found to be successful from published results by several authors. Early reports have demonstrated good to excellent improvements in clinical outcomes. Studies over the last decade have continued to provide evidence supporting the use of supramalleolar osteotomies for distal tibial varus and valgus deformities. **Table 3** reviews the current literature on supramalleolar osteotomies.

COMPLICATIONS

Complications from supramalleolar osteotomies have been reported as rare. Wound healing complications and infections have an incidence reported of up to 22%. Malunion or nonunion also has a complication of up to 22%. There is little evidence of surgical technique, use of allograft versus autograft, or type of fixation that yields best union rates in distal tibial osteotomies. The progression of degenerative OA after a supramalleolar osteotomy of the ankle joint was reported to be up to 25% in the literature. Progression of arthritis and pain can be treated with ankle arthrodesis or total ankle replacement successfully.

SUMMARY

Overall, supramalleolar osteotomy has been shown to have good midterm results in patients with midstage asymmetric ankle joint arthritis and varus or valgus distal tibial deformity. Studies have shown it is an effective option in avoiding joint-destructive ankle arthritis procedures. With proper patient selection and preoperative planning, the supramalleolar osteotomy can effectively redistribute the forces placed on the ankle, limiting progression of further degenerative changes and improve pain and functionality.

REFERENCES

1. Kimizuka M, Kurosawa H, Fukubayashi T. Load-bearing pattern of the ankle joint. Contact area and pressure distribution. Arch Orthop Trauma Surg 1980;96:45–9.
2. Valderrabano V, Horisberger M, Russell I, et al. Etiology of ankle osteoarthritis. Clin Orthop Relat Res 2009;467(7):1800–6.
3. Horisberger M, Valderrabano V, Hintermann B. Posttraumatic ankle osteoarthritis after ankle-related fractures. J Orthop Trauma 2009;23(1):60–7.
4. Ogilvie-Harris DJ, Sekyi-Otu A. Arthroscopic debridement for the osteoarthritic ankle. Arthroscopy 1995;11(4):433–6.
5. Saltzman CL, Hillis SL, Stolley MP, et al. Motion versus fixed distraction of the joint in the treatment of ankle osteoarthritis: a prospective randomized controlled trial. J Bone Joint Surg Am 2012;94(11):961–70.
6. Wiewiorski M, Barg A, Valderrabano V. Cartilage reconstruction in osteochondral lesions of the talus (OCLT). Foot Ankle Clin 2013. in press.
7. Tanaka Y. The concept of ankle joint preserving surgery: why does supramalleolar osteotomy work and how to decide when to do an osteotomy or joint replacement. Foot Ankle Clin 2012;17(4):545–53.
8. Ahmad J, Raikin SM. Ankle arthrodesis: the simple and the complex. Foot Ankle Clin 2008;13(3):381–400.
9. Barg A, Knupp M, Henninger HB, et al. Total ankle replacement using HINTEGRA, an unconstrained, three-component system: surgical technique and pitfalls. Foot Ankle Clin 2012;17(4):607–35.
10. Valderrabano V, Pagenstert GI, Müller AM, et al. Mobile- and fixed-bearing total ankle prostheses: is there really a difference? Foot Ankle Clin 2012;17(4):565–85.

11. Knupp M, Bolliger L, Hintermann B. Treatment of posttraumatic varus ankle deformity with supramalleolar osteotomy. Foot Ankle Clin 2012;17(1):95–102.
12. Speed JS, Boyd HB. Operative reconstruction of malunited fractures about the ankle joint. J Bone Joint Surg Am 1936;18(2):270–86.
13. Dzakhov SD, Kurochkin I. Supramalleolar osteotomies in children and adolescents. Ortop Travmatol Protez 1966;27(12):41–8.
14. Barskii AV, Semenov NP. Methods of the supramalleolar osteotomy in ununited fractures of the malleoli. Ortop Travmatol Protez 1979;7:54–5.
15. Takakura Y, Tanaka Y, Kumai T, et al. Low tibial osteotomy for osteoarthritis of the ankle. Results of a new operation in 18 patients. J Bone Joint Surg Br 1995;77(1):50–4.
16. Tarr RR, Resnick CT, Wagner KS. Changes in tibiotalar joint contact areas following experimentally induced tibial angular deformities. Clin Orthop 1985;199:72–80.
17. Kristensen KD, Kiaer T, Blicher J. No arthrosis of the ankle 20 years after maligned tibial shaft fracture. Acta Orthop Scand 1989;60:208–9.
18. Sammarco GJ. Biomechanics of the foot. In: Nordin M, Frankel VH, editors. Basic biomechanics of the musculoskeletal system. 2nd edition. Philadelphia: Lea & Febiger; 1989. p. 163.
19. Inman VT. The joints of the ankle. Baltimore (MD): Williams and Wilkins; 1976.
20. Paley D. Ankle and foot considerations. In: Paley D, editor. Principles of deformity correction. New York: Springer; 2002. p. 46, 572, 573, 581.
21. Weatherall JM, Mroczek K, McLaurin T, et al. Post-traumatic ankle arthritis. Bull Hosp Jt Dis 2013;71(1):104–12.
22. Giannini S, Buda R, Faldini C, et al. The treatment of severe posttraumatic arthritis of the ankle joint. J Bone Joint Surg Am 2007;89:15–28.
23. Rammelt S, Zwipp H. Intra-articular osteotomy for correction of malunions and nonunions of the tibial pilon. Foot Ankle Clin 2016;21(1):63–76.
24. Krause F, Veljkovic A, Schmid T. Supramalleolar osteotomies for posttraumatic malalignment of the distal tibia. Foot Ankle Clin 2016;21(1):1–14.
25. Paley D. Ankle malalignment. In: Kelikian A, editor. Operative treatment of the foot and ankle. Stamford (CT): Appleton & Lange; 1999. p. 547–86.
26. Barg A, Saltzman CL. Single-stage supramalleolar osteotomy for coronal plane deformity. Curr Rev Musculoskelet Med 2014;7:277–91.
27. Mangone PG. Distal tibial osteotomies for the treatment of foot and ankle disorders. Foot Ankle Clin 2001;6:583–97.
28. Mulhern JL, Protzman NM, Brigido SA. Supramalleolar osteotomy indications and surgical techniques. Foot Ankle Clin 2015;32(3):445–61.
29. Rush SM. Supramalleolar osteotomy. Clin Podiatr Med Surg 2009;26:245–57.
30. Mendicino RW, Catanzariti AR, Reeves CL. Percutaneous supramalleolar osteotomy for distal tibial (near articular) ankle deformities. J Am Podiatr Med Assoc 2005;95:72–84.
31. Myerson MS, Zide JR. Management of varus ankle osteoarthritis with joint-preserving osteotomy. Foot Ankle Clin 2013;18:471–80.
32. DiDomenico LA, Gatalyak N. End-stage ankle arthritis: arthrodiastasis, supramalleolar osteotomy, or arthrodesis? Clin Podiatr Med Surg 2012;29:391–412.
33. Stamatis ED, Myerson MS. Supramalleolar osteotomy: indications and technique. Foot Ankle Clin 2003;8:317–33.
34. Galli M, Scott R. Supramalleolar osteotomies an algorithm for the deformed ankle. Clin Podiatr Med Surg 2015;32(3):435–44.

35. Pagenstert GI, Hintermann B, Barg A, et al. Realignment surgery as alternative treatment of varus and valgus ankle osteoarthritis. Clin Orthop Relat Res 2007; 462:156–68.

36. Hintermann B, Knupp M, Barg A. Osteotomies of the distal tibia and hindfoot for ankle realignment. Orthopade 2008;37(3):212–3.

37. Gessmann J, Seybold D, Baecker H, et al. Correction of supramalleolar deformities with the Taylor spatial frame. Z Orthop Unfall 2009;147(3):314–20.

38. Hintermann B, Barg A, Knupp M. Corrective supramalleolar osteotomy for malunited pronation-external rotation fractures of the ankle. J Bone Joint Surg Br 2011;93(10):1367–72.

39. Knupp M, Stufkens SA, Bolliger L, et al. Classification and treatment of supramalleolar deformities. Foot Ankle Int 2011;32:1023–31.

40. Lee WC, Moon JS, Lee K, et al. Indications for supramalleolar osteotomy in patients with ankle osteoarthritis and varus deformity. J Bone Joint Surg Am 2011; 93(13):1243–8.

41. Knupp M, Barg A, Bolliger L, et al. Reconstructive surgery for overcorrected clubfoot in adults. J Bone Joint Surg Am 2012;94(15):e1101-7.

42. Barg A, Paul J, Pagenstert GI, et al. Supramalleolar osteotomies for ankle osteoarthritis. Tech Foot Ankle 2013;12:138–46.

43. Colin F, Bolliger L, Horn LT, et al. Effect of supramalleolar osteotomy and total ankle replacement on talar position in the varus osteoarthritic ankle: a comparative study. Foot Ankle Int 2014;35(5):445–52.

Osteochondral Autograft and Allograft Transplantation in the Talus

Alan Ng, DPM[a,b,*], Kaitlyn Bernhard, DPM[a]

KEYWORDS

- Osteochondral autograft transplantation ● Osteochondral allograft transplantation
- Hyaline articular cartilage ● Medial malleolar osteotomy ● OATS

KEY POINTS

- Large, symptomatic, focal chondral, and osteochondral lesions of the ankle have been treated over the past 15 years with osteochondral autograft/allograft transplantation (OAT) procedure.
- The OAT procedure is a reconstructive bone grafting technique that uses one or more cylindrical osteochondral grafts from an area of low impact or allograft source and transplants them into the prepared defect site on the talus.
- Performed through miniarthrotomy or malleolar osteotomy this technique allows defects to be filled with osteochondral plug with mature hyaline articular cartilage.
- Acute or chronic chondral or osteochondral lesions can be a debilitating condition, especially in the younger athletic population; provided here is a review of osteochondral autograft or allograft transplantation.
- OAT procedure shows successful outcomes for large osteochondral lesions or for revision osteochondral defect repair.

INTRODUCTION

Large, symptomatic, focal chondral, or osteochondral lesions of the ankle have been treated over the past 15 years with osteochondral autograft/allograft transplantation (OAT) procedure.[1-3] The surgical technique was first described for treating lesions in the knee by Yamashita and colleagues in 1985.[4] Improvements on the procedure continued over the next decade while Hangody and Fules popularized the modern technique.[5] Performed via open, miniarthrotomy, or arthroscopic-assisted approaches, this technique allows defects to be filled immediately with mature, hyaline articular cartilage.[6] Ideally, a cylindrical plug of healthy cartilage and subchondral

[a] PMSR/RRA, Highlands/Presbyterian St. Luke's Podiatric Surgical Residency Program, 1719 East 19th Avenue, Denver, CO 80218, USA; [b] Private Practice, Advanced Orthopedic and Sports Medicine Specialists, 8101 East Lowry Boulevard #230, Denver, CO 80230, USA
* Corresponding author. PMSR/RRA, Highlands/Presbyterian St. Luke's Podiatric Surgical Residency Program, 1719 East 19th Avenue, Denver, CO 80218.
E-mail address: ankleftdoc@aol.com

Clin Podiatr Med Surg 34 (2017) 461–469
http://dx.doi.org/10.1016/j.cpm.2017.05.004
0891-8422/17/© 2017 Elsevier Inc. All rights reserved.

bone is harvested from an area of low impact. Depending on the size of the lesion, mosaicplasty could afford a better fit, utilizing multiple smaller sized plugs to fill the defect. Acute or chronic chondral or osteochondral lesions can be a debilitating condition, especially in the younger athletic population; provided here is a review of osteochondral autograft or allograft transplantation.

CLINICAL PRESENTATION

A typical clinical presentation of osteochondral lesion of the talus (OLT) includes symptoms such as pain, mechanical locking, and catching of the ankle joint with range of motion. A single injury or multiple traumatic events can result in some form of cartilage injury. Approximately one-half of acute ankle sprains are likely to cause chondral or osteochondral pathology.[7] In addition, a study reviewed 84 acute ankle fractures, and of those fractures, 61 (73%) had concomitant chondral injuries.[8] Those individuals describing deep ankle pain with weight bearing, impaired function, stiffness, and even swelling raise clinical suspicion for ankle joint pathology.[9] A diagnostic ankle block helps differentiate between ankle joint pain and extra-articular pathology, while providing therapeutic benefits for the patient.

INDICATIONS/CONTRAINDICATIONS

OAT procedures are primarily reserved for larger, (>1 cm^2), isolated lesions and subchondral cystic lesions of the talus.[10] If the primary treatment for smaller defects fails to resolve with excision, debridement, and bone marrow stimulation, then the OAT procedure should be considered.[9] OLTs secondary to avascular necrosis have been shown to be at higher risk for failure because of the decreased vascularity resulting in poor incorporation of the graft.[2] With autograft transplantation, it is not recommended to treat a defect greater than 4 cm^2 due to donor site morbidity.[5] Some contraindications include infection, inflammatory arthropathy, neuropathy, vascular disease, degenerative joint disease of the tibiotalar joint, uncorrectable malalignment, and ligamentous instability.[11] Lesions of the talar shoulder are also a relative contraindication.

IMAGING PREPARATION

Subtle findings can be detected on plain radiographs, with up to 50% to 66% of OLT appearing as trabecular bone irregularities.[12] It is helpful to obtain ankle radiographs of anterior-posterior, lateral, and mortise views to clearly demonstrate the talar dome.[10] In cases with normal radiographs but high clinical suspicion, advanced imaging such as computed tomography (CT) and magnetic resonance imagining (MRI) may be performed to make a more definitive diagnosis. MRI has certain advantages over CT, being able to demonstrate bone marrow edema and the stability of the OLT. However, MRI is less precise in bone analysis compared with CT. Specifically, CT-arthrogram is superior to both with its ability to demonstrate precise analysis of the bone matrix and the cartilaginous cover provided by arthrography.[10] Although bone scintigraphy does not provide a definitive diagnosis, it remains useful in the exploration of unexplained pain. Intraoperative arthroscopy provides the most accurate diagnosis, when prior imaging may have misinterpreted the findings. As with each imaging modality, classification systems have been developed to better understand the progression of the lesion (**Table 1**).

TECHNIQUE

A key principle for the OAT procedure to be successful is to have perpendicular access for both plug harvest and transfer. A distal fibular osteotomy can be utilized for

Table 1
Proposed classification schemes of OLTs based on imaging modalities

	Stage 1	Stage 2a	Stage 2b	Stage 3	Stage 4	Stage 5
Radiograph	Subchondral bone compression	Partially detached osteochondral fragment	N/A	Detached fragment, remains in place	Displaced fragment	Subchondral cyst formation
MRI	Trabecular compression	Subchondral cysts	Non-detached fragment	Non-displaced fragment	Displaced fragment	
CT	Subchondral cyst but intact joint surface	Subchondral cyst with open cartilage	Open cartilage, non-displaced fragment	Subchondral cyst, non-displaced fragment	Displaced fragment	
Arthroscopy Note: Does not follow above stages	(A) Soft, smooth cartilage	(B) Rough cartilage	(C) Fibrillation and fissures	(D) Flap or naked bone	(E) Sequestrum in place	(F) Displaced fragment

Data from Refs.[25–28]

lateral talar dome lesions. Plafondplasty provides access to the anterior 75% of the talus with plantarflexion.[13] For medial talar dome lesions, the lesions can be reached with a medial malleolar osteotomy (**Figs. 1–3**). A study by Bull and colleagues[14] retrospectively reviewed 50 biplane medial malleolar chevron osteotomies fixated with 2 lag screws and demonstrated a 30% malunion rate with an average of 2 mm of incongruence on radiographs. From their results, they have implemented a distal tibia medial buttress plate in addition to the 2 parallel screw construct to reduce postoperative osteotomy displacement. Malleolar osteotomies allow for perpendicular access; however, an osteotomy displacement can result in local ankle arthritis.

For autologous harvest, sites should be located at nonweight-bearing portions such as the intercondylar notch and medial or lateral femoral condyles of the knee. The plantar and medial aspect of the talar head is another option for foot and ankle surgeons. Although osteochondral allograft eliminates donor site complications, there remains a low but nonzero risk of infectious disease transmission. Osteochondral allografts can be divided into 3 groups, consisting of freeze-dried, fresh-frozen, and fresh, cold-stored. Viable chondrocytes are best preserved in the fresh, cold-stored group. Cell viability, chondrocytes, and extracellular matrix of the mature articular cartilage decrease by only 1.7% after 14 days, but 28.5% after 28 days.[13] Whether autograft or allograft is used for the osteochondral plug, it is critical for the graft to be inserted flush with the surrounding articular surface (**Figs. 4–6**). Animal studies have shown that a graft countersunk greater than 2 mm will undergo cartilage necrosis and fibrous overgrowth, while a graft left proud demonstrates micromotion in its bed and fissuring of its hyaline cartilage.[15] There are varying differences of average cartilage thickness for the talus, femur, patella, and tibial plateau, which are 0.89, 2.0, 3.33, and 2.92 mm, respectively.[12] Talar autograft or allografts may be a better option for OLT to achieve anatomic congruency with regards to cartilage thickness.

After preoperative planning of which harvest graft would be best for the patient, the OAT procedure can proceed. Arthroscopy can be performed first utilizing standard anteromedial and anterolateral portals to assess the size and location of the lesion. If arthroscopy is not an option, then an open or mini arthrotomy can be utilized, as well, in order to visualize the ankle joint. After inspecting the ankle joint for any other pathology, the osteochondral lesion is identified, and the surrounding cartilage is inspected using a probe. Excision and debridement are done to prepare the recipient site by establishing a healthy, stable articular rim around the defect and for accurate measurement of the lesion.

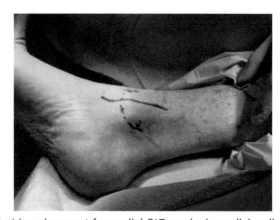

Fig. 1. Surgical incision placement for medial OLT repair via medial malleolar osteotomy.

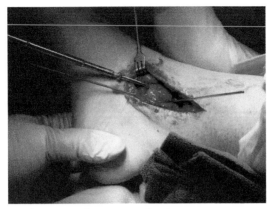

Fig. 2. Pre-osteotomy placement of osteotomy hardware.

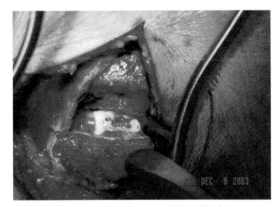

Fig. 3. Osteochondral lesion of the talus after medial malleolar osteotomy.

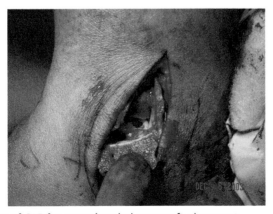

Fig. 4. Preparation of OLT for osteochondral autograft placement.

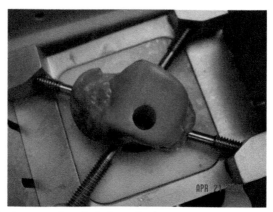

Fig. 5. Harvest of talar osteochondral allograft plug.

Next, it is important to proceed with the donor harvest, autograft or allograft, before drilling the recipient site. If using autograft, the donor graft harvest site should be easily accessible with minimal morbidity. With the cylindrical harvester seated to the articular cartilage firmly, a manual technique should be used to reduce the risk of thermal necrosis and adverse effects on the viable chondrocytes. Access to the Osteochondral lesion is then performed through malleolar arthrotomy or plafondplasty. The authors preferred technique is typically a oblique medial malleolar osteotomy to access lesions on the medial half of the talus and an oblique osteotomy of fibula for lateral lesions. As visualized in **Fig. 2**, the osteotomy is planned with a kirschner wire and visualized under fluoroscopy to ensure the osteotomy is placed in the proper orientation. Pre-placement of screws is accomplished prior to osteotomy to ensure anatomic reduction. The author prefers complete insertion of screws rather than only pre-drilling of holes to ensure anatomic reduction when fixation of the osteotomy is performed. When definitive fixation is placed, it is common for the screw length to increase by 5 mm in order to ensure solid screw purchase in native bone. The recipient site is then drilled to the same depth and diameter as that of the harvested plug, ensuring that the base has a stable vascularized zone in order to both potentiate vascular ingrowth for incorporation of the graft and to promote healing of fibrocartilage between plugs when used with mosaicplaty. The graft should be pressed fit with digital

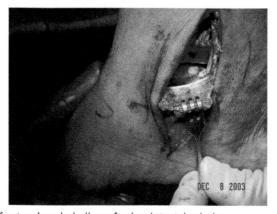

Fig. 6. Press fit of osteochondral allograft plug into talar lesion.

pressure. If multiple plugs are utilized, a common pattern of insertion involves initially working peripherally, thus inserting the central plug last.[6]

FOLLOW-UP CARE

In cases of osteochondral allograft or talar autograft transplantation procedures, litera-ture recommends a range of three to 6 weeks of non-weightbearing with the use of a posterior splint for the first 2 weeks followed by a below knee case for the duration of the non weightbearing period. The initial non-weightbearing phase is recommended to prevent graft subsidence during osseous integration. Patients are then transitioned to a removable walking boot for protected weight bearing. Partial weightbearing supports fibrocartilage repair among implanted cylindrical plugs, further enhancing secure graft incorporation. A 6-week course of physical therapy, two visits per week, focusing on joint mobilizations, strength, and balance is initiated at 8 weeks. At approximately 3 months post-operatively, patients are fully transitioned into normal shoe gear[11,16,17] (**Fig. 7**).

As previously mentioned, one of the biggest adverse outcomes that can be had with this procedure is a malleolar malunion or non-union, which can occur because of dissection, procedure selection, hardware considerations, or improper follow-up. Several papers exist which state that tibial or fibular osteotomies to gain access to OLTs are safe and heal efficiently. A recent anatomic study showed that 62.5% of tibial osteotomies do not even violate cartilage at the transitional zone between the tibial plafond and the medial malleolus.[18] The same paper published findings in 17 patients who underwent medial malleolar osteotomy. They found all osteotomies healed within 3 months and only one patient had a visible step incongruency of the tibial plafond. Three additional patients had evidence of local joint degeneration. A review of 342 pa-tients who underwent medial malleolar osteotomy revealed a 2.3% complication rate,

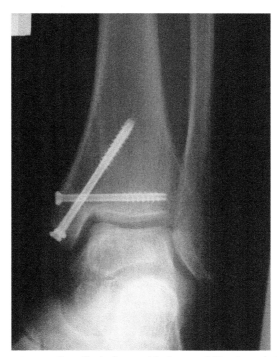

Fig. 7. 8 months post-operative, displaying multi-plane stabilization of the osteotomy.

including delayed union, non-union, broken or painful screws, and non-specific pain.[19] Still, care must be taken to prevent malleolar osteotomy complications after surgery. Several studies report much more complications, including osteoarthritic changes in 20% to 50% of patients at 5 years follow-up, while another study found cartilage damage in 29% of these cases via second look arthroscopy,[20–22] in addition to the previously discussed article from Bull.[14]

SUMMARY

The OAT procedure is a reconstructive bone grafting technique that uses one or more cylindrical osteochondral grafts from an area of low impact or allograft source and transplants them into the prepared defect site on the talus. Its goal is to reproduce the mechanical, structural, and biochemical properties of the original hyaline articular cartilage.[9] In 2001, Hangody evaluated the clinical outcomes of 36 patients that were followed for two to 7 years after a mosaicplasty with autogenous osteochondral transplantation from the knee to the ipsilateral talus. Ankle function was measured by the Hannover scoring system and showed good to excellent results in 34 cases (94%) with no long term donor site morbidity.[23] A larger study by Hangody a few years later included 1097 mosaicplasties, and of those 98 were performed for talar lesions. Analysis of clinical scores showed good to excellent results in 93% of talar dome procedures. Moderate and severe donor-site disturbances were present in 3% of patients. These patients were assessed by clinical evaluation and scoring with the Hannover and Bandi scoring systems.[16] In a systematic review, nine publications described the results of 243 patients treated by osteochondral transplantation. In 212 patients (87%) had good or excellent results. Donor knee morbidity was seen in 12% of patients (0%–37%), however, three studies did not investigate post-operative knee pain.[9] A study of thirty-eight patients underwent singular fresh osteochondral allograft plug for OLT that was greater than 2 cm². There was a 73% rate of good or excellent results at an average of 38 months.[24] Still, there remains a dearth of literature in regards to long term follow-up for this procedure; however, OAT shows a trend toward greater longevity and durability as well as improved outcomes in high-demand patients when compared to other options for osteochondral lesion repair.[6]

REFERENCES

1. Chang E, Lenczner E. Osteochondritis dissecans of the talar dome treated with an osteochondral autograft. Can J Surg 2000;43(3):217–21.
2. Gautier E, Kolker D, Jacob R. Treatment of cartilage defects of the talus by autologus osteochondral grafts. Bone Joint J 2002;84(2):237–44.
3. Hangody L. The mosaicplasty technique for osteochondral lesions of the talus. Foot Ankle Clin 2003;8(2):259–73.
4. Yamashita F, Sakakida K, Suzu F, et al. The transplantation of an autogenic osteochondral fragment for osteochondritis dissecans of the knee. Clin Orthop Relat Res 1985;(201):43–50.
5. Hangody L, Fules P. Autologous osteochondral mosaicplasty for the treatment of full-thickness defects of weight-bearing joints: ten years of experimental and clinical experience. J Bone Joint Surg Am 2003;85a(Suppl 2):25–32.
6. Richter DL, Tanksley JA, Miller MD. Osteochondral autograft transplantation: a review of the surgical technique and outcomes. Sports Med Arthrosc Rev 2016; 24(2):74–8.
7. Saxena A, Eakin C. Articular talar injuries in athletes: results of microfracture and autogenous bone graft. Am J Sports Med 2007;35(10):1680–7.

8. Leontaritis N, Hinojosa L, Panchbhavi V. Arthroscopically detected intra-articular lesions associated with acute ankle fractures. J Bone Joint Surg Am 2009;91(2):333–9.

9. Zengerink M, Struijs P, Tol J, et al. Treatment of osteochondral lesions of the talus: a systematic review. Knee surgery, sports traumatology. Arthroscopy 2010;18(2):238–46.

10. Laffenetre O. Osteochondral lesions of the talus: current concept. Orthop Traumatol Surg Res 2010;96(5):554–66.

11. Berlet G, Hyer C, Philbin T, et al. Does fresh osteochondral allograft transplantation of talar osteochondral defects improve function? Clin Orthop Relat Res 2011;469(8):2356–66.

12. Giza E. Operative techniques for osteochondral lesions of the talus. Foot Ankle Spec 2008;1(4):250–2.

13. Fuchs D. Osteochondral allograft transplantation in the ankle: a review of current practice. Orthop Res Rev 2015;7:95–105.

14. Bull P, Berlet G, Canini C, et al. Rate of malunion following bi-plane chevron medial malleolar osteotomy. Foot Ankle Int 2016;37(6):620–6.

15. Huang F, Simonian P, Norman A, et al. Effects of small incongruities in a sheep model of osteochondral autografting. Am J Sports Med 2004;32(8):1842–8.

16. Hangody L, Vasarhelyi G, Hangody L, et al. Autologous osteochondral grafting—technique and long-term results. Injury 2008;39(Suppl 1):532–9.

17. Mendeszoon M, Wilson N, Avramaut K, et al. Surgical correction of OCD utilizing OATS procedure harvested from head of the talus. North Ohio Foot Ankle J 2015;2(9):2.

18. Leumann A, Horisberger M, Buettner O, et al. Medial malleolar osteotomy for the treatment of talar osteochondral lesions: anatomical and morbidity considerations. Knee Surg Sports Traumatol Arthrosc 2016;24:2133–9.

19. Barg A, Pagenstert G, Leumann A, et al. Malleolar osteotomy–osteotomy as approach. Orthopade 2013;42(5):309–21.

20. MacCullough C, Venugopal V. Osteochondritis dissecans of the talus: the natural history. Clin Orthop Relat Res 1979;144:264–8.

21. Gaulrapp H, Hagena F, Wasmer G. Postoperative assessment of osteochondritis dissecans of the talus with special reference to Innenknöchelosteotomie. Z Orthop Unfall 1996;134(4):346–53 [in German].

22. Lee K, Kim J, Young K, et al. The use of fibrin matrix-mixed gel-type autologous chondrocyte implantation in the treatment for osteochondral lesions of the talus. Knee Surg Sports Traumatol Arthrosc 2013;21:1251–60.

23. Hangody L, Kish G, Modis L, et al. Mosaicplasty for the treatment of osteochondritis dissecans of the talus: two to seven year results in 36 patients. Foot Ankle Int 2001;22(7):552–8.

24. El-Rashidy H, Villacis D, Omar I, et al. Fresh osteochondral allograft for the treatment of cartilage defects of the talus: a retrospective review. J Bone Joint Surg 2011;93(17):1634–40.

25. Berndt A, Harty M. Transchondral fractures (osteochondritis dissecans) of the talus. J Bone Joint Surg Am 1959;41a:988–1020.

26. Anderson B, Crichton KJ. Osteochondral fractures of the dome of the talus. J Bone Joint Surg 1989;62A:1143–52.

27. Ferkel R, Sgaglione N, Pizzo WD. Arthroscopic treatment of osteochondral lesions of the talus: long-term results. Orthop Trans 1990;14:172–3.

28. Ferkel R. Arthroscopic surgery: the foot and ankle. Philadelphia: Lippincott Raven; 1996.

Advances in Ankle Cartilage Repair

Alan Ng, DPM[a,b,*], Andrew Bernhard, DPM[a,c], Kaitlyn Bernhard, DPM[a]

KEYWORDS

- Osteochondral lesion of talus • Allograft cartilage replacements
- Autograft cartilage replacements

KEY POINTS

- Repair of osteochondral lesions of the talus remains a hot topic due to the high incidence and troublesome long-term nature of these injuries.
- Smaller lesions will respond well to simple arthroscopy and microfracture, whereas larger cystic lesions may require allograft talus replacement or ankle fusions.
- The lesions in between are significantly more difficult to treat, with no gold standard currently in place. Autologous chondrocyte implantation and matrix-associated autologous chondrocyte implantation have been around for several years with promising results, whereas newer techniques and products, such as particulated juvenile allograft cartilage and micronized cartilage matrix, offer hope for future treatment options. Still other products, such as Subchondroplasty, seek to change the way pain associated with osteochondral and bone marrow lesions is considered.
- Future research may be aimed at new techniques, pharmacologic intervention, and cell-based therapies, and may be better served with prospective observational studies rather than costly randomized controlled studies.

INTRODUCTION

The ankle joint can be described as a near perfect joint. Unlike other large, loadbearing joints, the ankle rarely develops osteoarthritis unless there is some prior trauma. Once trauma occurs, however, ankle arthritis can become a significant source of morbidity. Primary ankle osteoarthritis (OA) in the absence of trauma accounts for only 7% to 9% of ankle arthritis, whereas up to 78% of cases are secondary to trauma.[1] No matter the cause, arthritis worsens quickly in the ankle joint because of the specialized nature of cartilage tissue and its inherent inability to regenerate.[2] Cartilage repair and regeneration techniques seek to prevent arthritis before bony adaptation can occur, in an

[a] PMSR/RRA, Highlands/Presbyterian St. Luke's Podiatric Surgical Residency Program, 1719 East 19th Avenue, Denver, CO 80218, USA; [b] Private Practice, Advanced Orthopedic and Sports Medicine Specialists, 8101 East Lowry Boulevard #230, Denver, CO 80230, USA; [c] Private Practice, Eagle-Summit Foot & Ankle, 50 Buck Creek Road #205, Avon, CO 81620, USA
* Corresponding author. PMSR/RRA, Highlands/Presbyterian St. Luke's Podiatric Surgical Residency Program, 1719 East 19th Avenue, Denver, CO 80218.
E-mail address: ankleftdoc@aol.com

Clin Podiatr Med Surg 34 (2017) 471–487
http://dx.doi.org/10.1016/j.cpm.2017.05.005
0891-8422/17/© 2017 Elsevier Inc. All rights reserved.

attempt to prevent larger, more debilitating surgeries, such as ankle arthrodesis or implant arthroplasty.

Arthroscopic interventions have long been the gold standard of osteochondral lesions of the talus (OLT) and can include bone marrow stimulation, retrograde drilling, and even osteochondral autograft transportation, which are outside of the scope of this article. Newer techniques for ankle cartilage repair still include cartilage autografts, such as autologous chondrocyte implantation (ACI) and matrix-associated ACI (MACI); allograft tissues, such as particulated juvenile allograft cartilage (PJAC); and cartilage matrices. Though initial research for ACI and MACI goes back decades in both the knee and ankle, the techniques are still among the more novel approaches. Allograft cartilage replacements have begun to replace these autogenous processes because they have similar results and only necessitate one surgery for the patient. The most researched of these is the class of PJAC, with DeNovo NT (Zimmer-Biomet, Warsaw, IN, USA), the most recognized brand name, supplying allogeneic chondrocytes to the chondral defect. Other newer cartilage matrices, such as BioCartilage (Arthrex, Naples, FL, USA), are used in conjunction with marrow stimulation and act as an extracellular matrix or scaffold for chondrocytes to thrive.

Finally, the state of future developments is discussed. Several articles have been written in the last 2 years discussing the lack of new basic research being done on cartilage regeneration. Specifically, talar cartilage defects and the associated treatments cannot simply be extrapolated from research done in other body parts due to the unique nature of cartilage in the ankle joint.[3] Cell-based therapies, such as multipotent stem cells and amniotic grafts, disease-modifying OA drugs, and joint distraction for intrinsic cartilage repair are future courses of treatment that may prove beneficial with more research.[4]

PERTINENT ANATOMY

Hyaline cartilage of the ankle joint, and notably the talus, is different than cartilage seen elsewhere in the body. The cells and matrix constituents are the same; however, it behaves differently with decreased thickness, response to insult, and vulnerability to injury.[3] The ankle is a synovial hinge joint, with 3 bones articulating. The articular surfaces of the talus, tibia, and fibula show more congruency than that of the tibia and femur in the knee.[5] The articular surface of the knee shows more variability in the thickness of cartilage, as well as increased thickness as a whole. Mean ankle cartilage thickness ranges from 1 to 1.7 mm thick, whereas the knee ranges from 1.5 to 6 mm thick, depending on location.[6,7] All of these differences highlight that small deviations in ankle anatomy predispose the ankle to osteochondral defects and arthritis.

The question of why osteochondral lesions are painful has recently been revisited. Van Dijk and colleagues[8] published a review suggesting that pain is caused by joint fluid forced underneath cartilage, into subchondral bone. This was also suggested to cause cyst formation within the talus. Before this occurs, however, persistent bone marrow edema is noted. Bone marrow lesions (BMLs) are thought to be associated with pain because they represent a healing response to underlying trauma and trabecular injury.[9] Talar cartilage, being thinner than knee cartilage, has also been shown to be less elastic and almost 50% of articular cartilage undergoes more than 15% of contact strain with normal weightbearing.[10] This combination of increased pressure across the joint, with decreased elasticity of the cartilage may lead to painful osteochondral lesions.

AUTOGRAFT CARTILAGE REPLACEMENTS

One of the earliest treatment options for osteochondral lesion repair was the osteochondral autograft transplant, developed by Yamashita and colleagues[11] in the late 1970s. His technique involved harvesting large nonweightbearing osteochondral segment that was largely nonarticular. The technique was retooled for talar lesions with Hangody and colleagues[12] publishing results on mosaicplasty with knee cartilage harvest by 1997. (See Alan Ng and Kaitlyn Bernhard's article, "Osteochondral Autograft and Allograft Transplantation in the Talus," in this issue.)

More recently, 2-stage procedures involving harvesting of chondral tissue, subsequent culture, and reimplantation have been described with great results. ACI and MACI are similar techniques that function via cell culture, to help induce cartilage formation at the site of the cartilaginous defect. The original description was, again, in the knee and developed in the 1980s.[13] Since then, MACI has largely replaced ACI because the matrix integration with the cartilage culture provides a built-in scaffold for cartilage growth and decreases the need for periosteal flap coverage of the deficit. These procedures remain elusive in the United States because they lack US Food and Drug Administration (FDA) approval and are generally not reimbursed financially. Indications, as elucidated in a recent review, for autogenous chondrocyte implantation as a whole includes any lesion requiring revisional surgery, lesions greater than 1.5 cm^2, cystic lesions, patients between 15 and 55 years old, a lack of arthritis or kissing lesions, and the absence of instability and malalignment. Following these guidelines, the investigators saw formation of hyaline and fibrocartilage at the site of the lesion with no formation of fibrous tissue. Their average subjects had lesions of 185 mm^2 and 193 mm^2 for ACI and MACI, respectively. All postoperative measurements, using the Mazur ankle score, were significantly improved in both groups at an average of 4.6 and 6.8 years for the respective procedures.[14]

The surgical technique for both procedures is comparable, with the first stage being identical. The initial surgical intervention involves standard ankle arthroscopy with full evaluation of the ankle joint. Anterolateral and anteromedial portals are achieved and the full 21-point examination of Stetson and Ferkel[15] is performed, with specific identification of the chondral lesion noted. For lesions that are difficult to reach, noninvasive ankle joint distraction can aid with visualization of the defect. The chondral lesion is debrided of any nonviable tissue, including cartilage and subchondral bone; if there is an osteochondral fragment that can be removed in total, it can be used for culture.[16] If this is not the case, a 10 by 3mm sample of cartilage is removed from the anterior aspect of the talar head.[14] This cartilage is then sent for culture of the chondrocytes.

The second surgery is where the 2 techniques diverge. After 3 to 4 weeks, the newly cultured cartilage is ready to be reimplanted. In ACI, this process generally requires an open procedure via tibia or fibula osteotomy, followed by fresh re-examination of the osteochondral lesion. The lesion is, again, debrided, down to healthy subchondral bone. If subchondral cystic changes are noted, the deficit will need to be packed before application of the cartilage graft. This can be allograft or autograft bone and just enough to fill the deficit. The chondrocytes are placed within a bilayer of harvested periosteum from the tibia, traditionally,[14] or a scaffold, as advocated by Giannini and colleagues,[17] and fastened with fibrin glue in a dry field.

The advantage of MACI is there is no need for a secondary scaffold or periosteal flap, as well as fixation of the graft. During the culture stage of the technique, new cartilage cells are grown on a matrix of type I and III collagen. The graft is able to be fixated with only fibrin glue. Without suture, the cartilage is able to return to a more hyaline-like state.[18]

Results have been promising for ACI and MACI, due to the newer nature of the procedure, though high-quality studies are still lacking. One large meta-analysis provides good insight into autograft transplantation results as a whole. Sixteen studies were identified in this 2011 review, covering 213 cases. Of note, only 6 of the 16 studies were actually ACI; the remaining 10 used MACI techniques, including Hyalograft C (Anika Therapeutics S.r.l., Padova, Italy), Chondrosphere (Regenerative Medical System, Seoul, Korea), and Chondron (co.don AG, Berlin, Germany). The overall clinical success rate was shown to be 89.9% at 32 months for defects averaging 2.3 cm^2.[19] Since then, a newer systemic review of ACI techniques, again evaluating both ACI and MACI side by side, has been published. Now, 19 articles meet inclusion criteria, with 6 studies demonstrating arthroscopic MACI, 8 performing open MACI, and 5 studies using ACI. The overall evidence level was low; however, they did conclude that American Orthopedic Foot and Ankle Society Score (AOFAS) was improved in open versus arthroscopic MACI, though open MACI had significantly more complications.[20]

ALLOGRAFT CARTILAGE REPLACEMENTS

Allograft repairs for osteochondral defects have, historically, been saved for large cystic lesions or those on the talar shoulder, which both present difficulties for other OLT repair techniques. Using fresh, cadaver allografts allows for a matched specimen, so size and shape of the lesion are of little importance. Initially described in 2001, the procedure allowed for two-thirds of lesions greater than 1 cm in diameter to remain intact at 11 years of follow-up.[21] The remaining cases required fusion after resorption of the graft. The largest study to date has a sample size of 38 subjects, who underwent allograft talus replacement with plug-shaped allografts. Only 73% of subjects had good to excellent results at an average of 38 months.[22] Because of the large, difficult nature of these lesions, ankle fusion or replacement often remains the gold standard of treatment.

Recently, however, allograft cartilage has taken on a new meaning entirely. PJAC is a new class of tissue consisting of exactly what it says, morselized cartilage fragments from cadaveric cartilage of donors less than 13 years old. The only product currently on the market is DeNovo NT, which is obtained from donors generally less than 13 years old. The graft is chondroconductive, chondroinductive, and chondrogenic but does, technically, incur the possibility of disease transmission due to the minimal manipulation it undergoes.[23] Indications are similar to those in ACI and MACI because the product is a cartilage graft. These include symptomatic OLTs larger than 15 mm in diameter, revision osteochondral defect repair, and lesions involving the shoulder of the talus.[24] The main contraindications include degenerative arthritic changes and a history of infection, along with a relative contraindication of large cystic lesions, which could require an osteochondral allograft. This last point is relative in that cystic lesions can often be treated with grafting of the cystic lesion with cancellous chips or structural bone graft, followed by placement of PJAC over the cartilaginous deficit.

The PJAC technique, originally described in the literature for the talus in 2010 and performed via an open ankle arthrotomy,[25] has already evolved in the few years it has been on the market. In 2012, an arthroscopic surgical technique was described, which the authors have been performing since 2008. After induction of anesthesia and obtaining a sterile field in the usual manner, a noninvasive ankle distractor is applied and the standard anteromedial and anterolateral portals are obtained. The OLT is debrided down to healthy subchondral bone using arthroscopic shavers and curettes, with care taken to ensure a sharp line of transition of healthy cartilage around the lesion. In cases in which the subchondral bone is not intact, the first layer of fibrin glue applied prevents the concern of bleeding of the cancellous bone, allowing the implant to take. The ankle joint is prepared for implantation by drying the joint with an abdominal insufflator and normal arthroscopic suction for at least 5 minutes. Once the subchondral bone of the OLT is dry, the cartilage graft is inserted through a 10-gauge catheter in the anteromedial portal onto a layer of fibrin glue. A second layer of fibrin glue is then applied over the cartilage to fill the remaining defect. The insufflator is, again, used to ensure the fibrin glue is dry to the touch before closing the arthroscopic portals.[26] A representative example of arthroscopic implantation can be followed in **Figs. 1–8**.

Because the product and techniques are new, long-term follow-up is still unavailable. A prospective study was published in 2014, however, evaluating the clinical and histologic success of PJAC for knee lesions.[27] They found statistically significant improvements in all measurements, including the International Knee Documentation Committee subjective and objective outcomes, the visual analog scale (VAS), and the Knee injury and Osteoarthritis Outcome Score at 2-year follow-up. Improvements from baseline were noted as early as 3 months postoperatively. A second-look procedure in 8 individuals revealed repair with a mix of hyaline and fibrocartilage, with increased type II cartilage identified. Very few researchers have studied PJAC in the talus, other than isolated case studies. With a follow-up of at least 12 months, one midterm study has results of 24 subjects who underwent this technique in the ankle. The study used retrospective enrollment and, as such, lacks preoperative baseline data. At 1 year, 1 delamination of the graft had occurred, whereas 6 of the subjects underwent a secondary procedure, none of which were related to the graft itself. For moderate lesions, 92% of subjects had a good or excellent outcome, with an AOFAS of more than 80, whereas only 56% of subjects with large lesions had similar results.[28]

BioCartilage is a separate, novel product consisting of dehydrated allogeneic cartilage chips that act as a scaffold or matrix for hyaline cartilage formation after microdrilling and debridement of OLTs. This product is the first in a class of micronized cartilage matrix (MCM) and contains proteoglycans and type II collagen, consistent

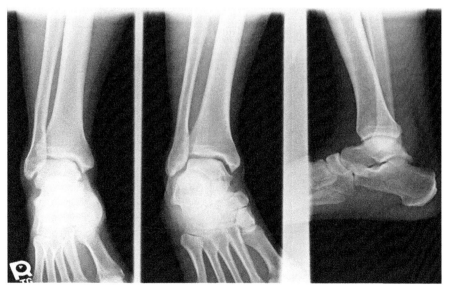

Fig. 1. A 26-year-old man with chief complaint of ankle pain.

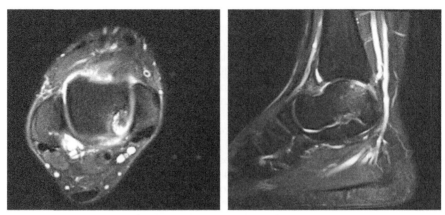

Fig. 2. Axial and sagittal MRI views showing posterolateral osteochondral lesion.

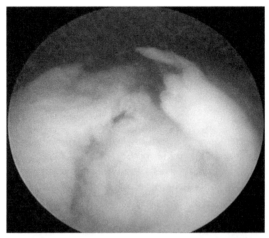

Fig. 3. OLT of the talar head before debridement.

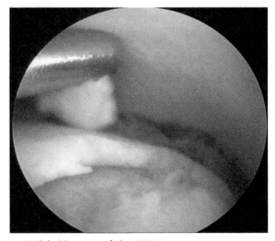

Fig. 4. Postarthroscopic debridement of the OLT.

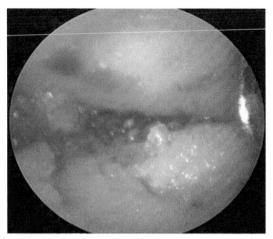

Fig. 5. Drying out of the ankle joint with insufflation.

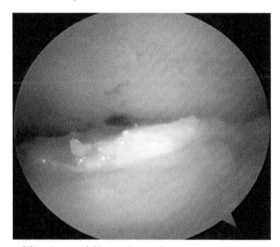

Fig. 6. Application of first layer of fibrin glue to bare OLT.

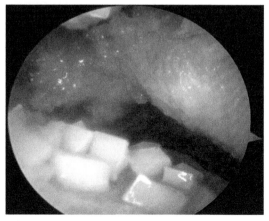

Fig. 7. Application of particulated juvenile allograft to fibrin glue.

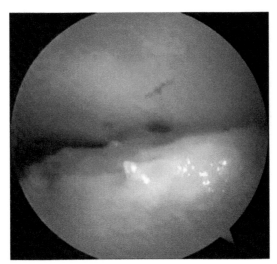

Fig. 8. Final application of fibrin glue over PJAC graft.

with hyaline cartilage formation. The operative technique also relies on platelet-rich plasma (PRP), to supply chondrogenic precursors and help sway differentiation.[29] The indications for this technique are similar to those of microfracture, which remains the core procedure performed at the authors' institution. These include smaller lesions, less than 15 mm in diameter or 150 mm^2 in surface area, noncystic lesions, and relative indications of less than 50 years and body mass index under 30. Contraindications include large cystic lesions, failure of multiple surgeries, and acute lesions for which there has been no attempt at conservative treatment. The operative technique is similar to microdrilling of chondral lesions, with the addition of harvest of bone marrow aspirate or PRP and application of the MCM. The OLT is debrided in the standard fashion, through arthroscopy with shavers and curettes, to a level of healthy subchondral bone and cartilage. Microfracture is also performed in a standard fashion with arthroscopic awls. The ankle joint is then evacuated and dried, as previously described for PJAC procedures. Any small cysts should be packed with harvested bone marrow aspirate or cancellous chips. The MCM and the bone marrow aspirate or PRP are mixed in a 1:1 ratio and applied to the OLT via injection through the arthroscopic portal. The remainder of the defect is coated with fibrin glue and allowed to dry for 5 minutes, with care taken to ensure the deficit is filled adequately and the cartilage is smooth.[30] The procedure can also be performed open if the OLT cannot be adequately visualized or prepared arthroscopically. A limited arthrotomy, or tibial or fibular osteotomy, may be necessary to apply the MCM, though the principles of applying dry and maintaining an even level with the surrounding cartilage remain.[31]

Results, not unlike the other techniques, are promising but require more studies. The technique report by Clanton and colleagues[30] offered results in a series of 7 subjects at an average of 8 months follow-up. Overall, subjects improved in all outcome measures, including all subscores of the Foot and Ankle Disability Index. A newer study discusses results from a case series of 22 subjects and used the Foot and Ankle Ability Measures and VAS scores for evaluation. At a mean of 20 months follow-up, there was statistical improvement in all outcome measurements. One subject required revisional osteochondral autograft/allograft transfer procedure at 6 months and another developed symptomatic degeneration of the ankle joint at 1 year.

SUBCHONDRAL BONE MARROW LESIONS

Some newer research is questioning why some osteochondral lesions are painful and others remain asymptomatic. One new technique, the Subchondroplasty (SCP) (Zimmer-Biomet, Warsaw, IN, USA), questions the paradigm of the pain emanating from the chondral lesion and instead presupposes that the pain is initiated by underlying bone marrow edema. The Van Dijk and colleagues[8] article, as previously discussed, suggests that intra-articular pressure forces joint fluid through the subchondral plate, resulting in subchondral cyst and BML formation. SCP involves buttressing the internal architecture of the BML, allowing it to heal with increased internal support.

Figs. 9 and **10** demonstrate a BML as an area of increased signal intensity on a T2-weighted MRI and an area of decreased signal intensity on T1-weighted MRI, respectively. A T2-weighted image may overestimate the true size of the BML, therefore it is important to correlate findings with a T1-weighted image. The surgeon should be cautious to not overfill the BML because too much bone substitute material may be painful for the patient. The technique involves arthroscopy of the ankle joint and identification of the osteochondral lesion and can be seen in **Figs. 11–18**. An injectable, synthetic calcium phosphate, AccuFill (Zimmer-Biomet, Warsaw, IN, USA) is inserted directly into the location of the BML under fluoroscopic guidance. The indications for this procedure are more related to the underlying BML, rather than the OLT itself. Ankle arthroscopy allows this to be directly visualized; the standard anterior portals are obtained to ensure that the subchondral bone plate is intact. Using fluoroscopy and the original MRI as reference, a cannula is inserted into the area of the BML, with care taken to correlate and triangulate positioning on true AP and lateral views. When the overlying cartilage and subchondral bone are intact, the cannula is inserted in a retrograde fashion. If subchondral bone plate is not intact, the cannula can be inserted anterograde directly into the lesion, as is seen in **Fig. 14** or it can be inserted in a retrograde fashion. Currently the authors preferred technique is to approach the lesion from a retrograde fashion to ensure the calcium phosphate is directed toward the failing subchondral bone. Anterograde approach can be utilized if the lesion is

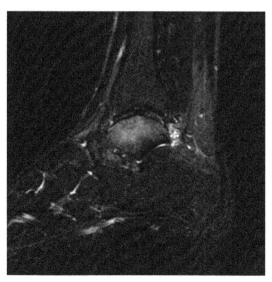

Fig. 9. BML on T2-weighted MRI with extensive bone marrow edema.

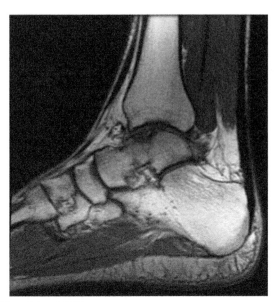

Fig. 10. BML on T1-weighted MRI.

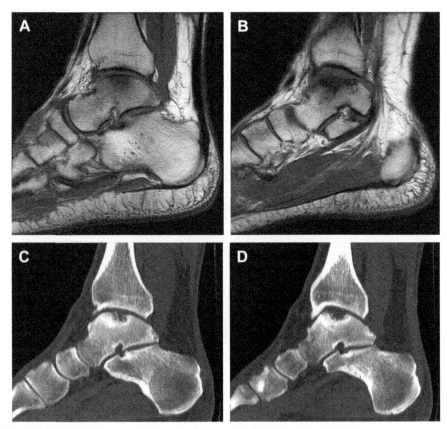

Fig. 11. (*A–D*) Initial presentation of a large central OLT on CT and MRI.

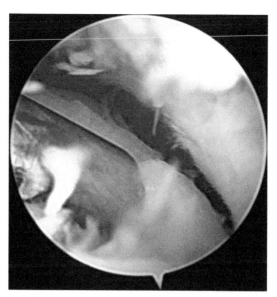

Fig. 12. Arthroscopic debridement of overlying diseased cartilage.

cystic to stabilize the subchondral bone beneath the ostochondral lesion. The AccuFill is injected directly into the lesion, creating a blush of the area on fluoroscopy, seen in **Fig. 15**. After 10 minutes of hardening time, all instrumentation is removed and arthroscopy is again performed to verify no extravasation has occurred,[32] as is the case in **Fig. 16**. This escaped calcium phosphate must be removed at the time of surgery. **Figs. 17** and **18** demonstrate how SCP can be used in conjunction with PJAC techniques. This allows the surgeon to address both the cartilaginous defect as well as the underlying BML, helping heal the microtrabecular injury and provide smooth, articular cartilage.

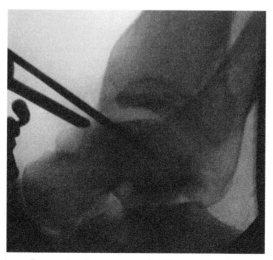

Fig. 13. Triangulation of cannula placement under fluoroscopy for SCP.

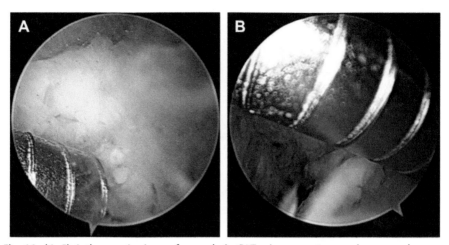

Fig. 14. (*A, B*) Arthroscopic views of cannula in OLT using an anterograde approach.

EMERGING CONCEPTS

Because no one technique has provided excellent long-term results, new approaches and products are continuing to be released and revised. A return to older procedures, such as microfracture surgery, with new techniques may prove valuable as well. Lift, drill, fill, and fix (LDFF) is a novel approach using the flapped chondral fragment as an autograft. Because of this, it is limited to those lesions in which the chondral fragment remains intact and is contraindicated when the flap is loose and floating. The procedure can be performed either arthroscopically or open, and requires subchondral drilling of the defect, followed by fixation of the overlying cartilage with a recessed

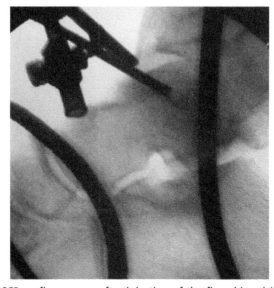

Fig. 15. Blush of SCP on fluoroscopy after injection of the flowable calcium phosphate.

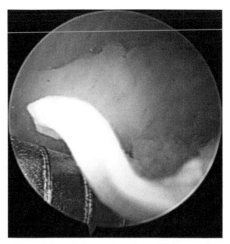

Fig. 16. Extravasation of flowable calcium phosphate. This needs to be removed with suction and the shaver.

absorbable compressive screw.[33] Results are promising, though lacking. One series of 9 subjects with 4 years follow-up had 78% good results and 22% fair results as reported with the Berndt-Harty clinical outcome scale.[34] A separate series of 7 subjects underwent arthroscopic LDFF and had AOFAS improve to 99 and pain numeric rating scale improve to 0.1 in a cohort of large, painful OLTs present for more than 1 year.[35]

Most of the techniques discussed here still lack long-term follow-up because of the novel approaches being used. Future products that may still prove effective include the Cartilage Autograft Implantation System (DePuy-Synthes, Raynham, MA, USA),

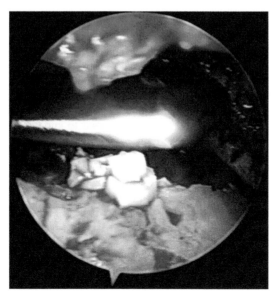

Fig. 17. Packing PJAC over the OLT defect after SCP application.

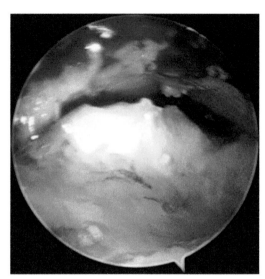

Fig. 18. Final appearance of lesion, in a dry scope, after application of last layer of fibrin glue.

which is similar to De Novo NT with autologous chondrocytes; Revaflex (ISTO Biologics, St. Louis, MO, USA), another PJAC; BST-CarGel (Smith & Nephew, Memphis, TN, USA), a bio-scaffold; and Novocart (Tetec, Reutlingen, Germany), a newer MACI. All of these are currently in registered FDA randomized controlled trials. Time will tell which of these techniques yields the greatest success rates.

Two major scientific publications have been negative about new developments in articular cartilage repairs in the last 3 years. A review in *Nature Reviews* suggests that significant improvements in inherent cartilage repair have not been achieved but 3 modalities offer promising futures. Disease-modifying osteoarthritic drugs offer the potential of preventing bone turnover and minimizing arthritic changes. No drugs are currently marketed as such; however, studies have looked at risedronate, doxycycline, and glucosamine and chondroitin supplementation in regard to joint space narrowing; with doxycycline, glucosamine, and chondroitin independently helping minimize joint space loss. Strontium has also been shown to aid cartilage matrix formation and stimulate chondrocyte proliferation. Cell-based therapies, such as MACI and De Novo NT implants, offer future potential as well (see previous discussion).[4] The final modality is joint distraction, which can lead to intrinsic functional repair of the underlying subchondral bone, even at 2 years postdistraction.[36]

The Journal of Bone and Joint Surgery published a forum earlier this year suggesting that cartilage repair is no longer moving forward and has been sluggish for the last 15 years due to regulations and costs associated with research. Specific mention is made of De Novo NT and BioCartilage as being approved as minimally treated grafts but, aside from these products, no new FDA-approved technologies have been seen since 1997. Several studies are underway, but they suggest that randomized controlled trials are too expensive and unwieldy to remain the approval criteria for new products. Cost, enrollment challenges, noncompliance, and equipoise all pose large problems to this type of research. The authors suggest that for the best new outcomes, other research designs should be supported, such as multicenter, prospective observational studies, as long as selection bias is able to be minimized.[37]

SUMMARY

Repair of OLT remains a hot topic due to the high incidence and troublesome long-term nature of these injuries. Many techniques currently exist and several treatment algorithms are available. Smaller lesions will respond well to simple arthroscopy and microfracture, whereas larger cystic lesions may require allograft talus replacement or ankle fusions. The lesions in between are significantly more difficult to treat, with no gold standard currently in place. ACI and MACI have been around for several years with promising results, whereas newer techniques and products, such as PJAC and MCM, offer hope for future treatment options. Still other products, such as SCP, seek to change the way pain associated with osteochondral and BMLs is considered. Future research may be aimed at new techniques, pharmacologic intervention, and cell-based therapies, and may be better served with prospective observational studies rather than costly randomized controlled studies.

REFERENCES

1. Valderrabano V, Horisberger M, Russell I, et al. Etiology of ankle arthritis. Clin Orthop Relat Res 2009;467(7):1800–6.
2. Anderson DD, Chubinskaya S, Guilak F, et al. Post-traumatic osteoarthritis: improved understanding and opportunities for early intervention. J Orthop Res 2011;29(6):802–9.
3. Anderson DD, Chubinskaya S, Guilak F, et al. Peculiarities in ankle cartilage. Cartilage 2017;8(1):12–8.
4. Mastbergen SC, Saris DB, Lafeber FP. Functional articular cartilage repair: here, near, or is the best approach not yet clear? Nat Rev Rheumatol 2013;9:277–90.
5. Hendren L, Beeson P. A review of the differences between normal and osteoarthritis articular cartilage in human knee and ankle joints. Foot (Edinb) 2009; 19(3):171–6.
6. Shepherd DE, Seedhom BB. Thickness of human articular cartilage in joints of the lower limb. Ann Rheum Dis 1999;58:27–34.
7. Millington SA, Grabner M, Wozelka Mag R, et al. Quantification of ankle articular cartilage topography and thickness using a high resolution stereophotography system. Osteoarthritis Cartilage 2007;15:205–11.
8. Van Dijk CN, Reilingh ML, Zengerink M, et al. Osteochondral defects in the ankle: why painful? Knee Surg Sports Traumatol Arthrosc 2010;18:570–80.
9. Eriksen EF, Ringe JD. Bone marrow lesions: a universal bone response to injury? Rheumatol Int 2012;32(3):575–84.
10. Wan L, de Asla RJ, Rubash HE, et al. In vivo cartilage contact deformation of human ankle joints under full body weight. J Orthop Res 2008;26:1081–9.
11. Yamashita F, Sakakida K, Suzu F, et al. The transplantation of an autogeneic osteochondral fragment for osteochondritis dissecans of the knee. Clin Orthop Relat Res 1985;201:43–50.
12. Hangody L, Kish G, Karpati Z, et al. Treatment of osteochondritis dissecans of the talus: use of the mosaicplasty technique—a preliminary report. Foot Ankle Int 1997;18(10):628–34.
13. Brittberg M, Lindahl A, Nilsson A, et al. Treatment of deep cartilage defects in the knee with autologous chondrocyte transplantation. N Engl J Med 1994;331(14): 889–95.
14. Johnson B, Lever C, Roberts S, et al. Cell cultured chondrocyte implantation and scaffold techniques for osteochondral talar lesions. Foot Ankle Clin 2013;18: 135–50.

15. Stetson WB, Ferkel R. Ankle arthroscopy: I. technique and complications. J Am Acad Orthop Surg 1996;4:17–23.
16. Giannini S, Buda R, Grigolo B, et al. The detached osteochondral fragment as a source of cells for autologous chondrocyte implantation (ACI) in the ankle joint. Osteoarthritis Cartilage 2005;13:601–7.
17. Giannini S, Buda R, Vannini F, et al. Arthroscopic autologous chondrocyte implantation in osteochondral lesions of the talus. Am J Sports Med 2008;36(5):873–80.
18. Ronga M, Grassi FA, Montoli C, et al. Treatment of deep cartilage defects of the ankle with matrix-induced autologous chondrocyte implantation (MACI). Foot Ankle Surg 2005;11:29–33.
19. Niemeyer P, Salzmann G, Schmal H, et al. Autologous chondrocyte implantation for the treatment of chondral and osteochondral defects of the talus: a meta-analysis of available evidence. Knee Surg Sports Traumatol Arthrosc 2012;20: 1696–703.
20. Gross CE, Erickson BJ, Fillingham YA, et al. Management of osteochondral lesions of the talus using autologous chondrocyte implantation: a systematic review. Foot & Ankle Orthopaedics 2016;1(1). [Epub ahead of print].
21. Gross AE, Agnidis Z, Hutchison CR. Osteochondral defects of the talus treated with fresh osteochondral allograft transplantation. Foot Ankle Int 2001;22(5): 385–91.
22. El-Rashidy H, Villacis D, Omar I, et al. Fresh osteochondral allograft for the treatment of cartilage defects of the talus: a retrospective review. J Bone Joint Surg Am 2011;93(17):1634–40.
23. Harris JD, Frank RM, McCormick FM, et al. Minced cartilage techniques. Operat Tech Orthop 2014;24:27–34.
24. Adams SB, Yao JQ, Schon LC. Particulated juvenile articular cartilage allograft transplantation for osteochondral lesions of the talus. Tech Foot Ankle Surg 2011;10(2):92–8.
25. Hatic SO, Berlet GC. Particulated juvenile articular cartilage graft (DeNovo NT Graft) for treatment of osteochondral lesions of the talus. Foot Ankle Spec 2010;3(6):361–4.
26. Kruse DL, Ng A, Paden M, et al. Arthroscopic De Novo NT juvenile allograft cartilage implantation in the talus: a case presentation. J Foot Ankle Surg 2012;51: 218–21.
27. Farr J, Tabet SK, Margerrison E, et al. Clinical, radiographic, and histological outcomes after cartilage repair with particulated juvenile articular cartilage: a 2-year prospective study. Am J Sports Med 2014;42(6):1417–25.
28. Coetzee JC, Giza E, Schon LC, et al. Treatment of osteochondral lesions of the talus with particulated juvenile cartilage. Foot Ankle Int 2013;34(9):1205–11.
29. Adams GD, Mall NA, Fortier LA, et al. BioCartilage: background and operative technique. Oper Tech Sports Med 2013;21:116–24.
30. Clanton TO, Johnson NS, Matheny LM. Use of cartilage extracellular matrix and bone marrow aspirate concentrate in treatment of osteochondral lesions of the talus. Tech Foot Ankle Surg 2014;13:212–20.
31. Mascarenhas R, Saltzman BM, Fortier LA, et al. BioCartilage: new frontiers in cartilage restoration. In: Cartilage e-Book. CIC Edizioni Internazionali; 2015. p. 183–93.
32. Miller JR, Dunn KW. Subchondroplasty of the ankle: a novel technique. Foot Ankle Online J 2015;8(1):7.
33. Reilingh ML, Kerkhoffs GMMJ. Lift, drill, fill and fix (LDFF): a cartilage preservation technique in osteochondral talar defects. Cartilage lesions of the ankle. Berlin: Springer; 2015.

34. Reilingh ML, Kerkhoffs GM, Telkamp CJ, et al. Treatment of osteochondral defects of the talus in children. Knee Surg Sports Traumatol Arthrosc 2014;22(9): 2243–9.
35. Kerkhoffs GMMJ, Reilingh ML, Gerards RM, et al. Lift, drill, fill and fix (LDFF): a new arthroscopic treatment for talar osteochondral defects. Knee Surg Sports Traumatol Arthrosc 2016;24(4):1265–71.
36. Intema F, Thomas TP, Anderson DD, et al. Subchondral bone remodeling is related to clinical improvement after joint distraction in the treatment of ankle osteoarthritis. Osteoarthritis Cartilage 2011;19(6):668–75.
37. Lyman S, Nakamura N, Cole BJ, et al. Cartilage-repair innovation at a standstill: methodologic and regulatory pathways to breaking free. J Bone Joint Surg Am 2016;98(15):e63.

Open Ankle Arthrodesis

Samuel S. Mendicino, DPM[a], Alexis L. Kreplick, DPM[a],*,
Jeremy L. Walters, DPM[b]

KEYWORDS

- Ankle fusion • Arthritis • Deformity • PTTD

KEY POINTS

- Open ankle arthrodesis remains the standard in the operative treatment of end-stage ankle arthritis, allowing patients to regain function while decreasing pain and discomfort to the affected limb.
- Successful ankle arthrodesis is multifaceted and requires consideration of concomitant deformities, careful dissection, thorough joint preparation, rigid fixation, and postoperative compliance.
- A variety of acceptable fixation constructs exist. Advancements in technology allow appropriate fixation and may include a combination of plates, screws, and external fixation.

INTRODUCTION
History

Arthrodesis is a surgical approach commonly used to address long-standing pain and deformity, arthritis, and dysfunction in the foot and ankle. Albert[1] initially described arthrodesis in 1879 as a knee and ankle fusion for children with neuromuscular disorders. Moving into the 1900s, arthrodesis was used in the ankle as a surgical correction for poliomyelitis. By the early 1950s, Charnley[2] described compression arthrodesis using external fixation devices for ankle fusions. The goals of Charnley's[2] ankle arthrodesis were to eliminate shear forces and fixate with close apposition of bony surfaces. Compression across the arthrodesis site proved to be a necessary step to improve union rates. However, Charnley's[2] surgical method used a transverse anterior approach. This method was purportedly a more amenable incisional approach for compression.[2] This incision and dissection resulted in the sacrifice of tendons and neurovascular structures at the anterior ankle. Despite reports that vascular compromise from the loss of the anterior tibial artery and anesthesia resulting from the

Disclosure: The authors have nothing to disclose.
[a] PMSR/RRA, West Houston Medical Center, 12121 Richmond Avenue, Suite 417, Houston, TX 77082, USA; [b] Department of Surgery, Sentara Medical Group, 2790 Godwin Boulevard, Suite 355, Suffolk, VA 23434, USA
* Corresponding author.
E-mail address: gtefresearch@gmail.com

transection of nerves were unfounded misconceptions of the transverse anterior approach,[2] this technique was abandoned.

The lateral incision became more popular because of the access to the fibula for autogenously derived bone graft as well as visualization of the tibiotalar joint.[3] With the recent improvements and popularity of total ankle arthroplasty there has been a renewed increase in anterior ankle incisions for arthrodesis in order to preserve the lateral malleolus for possible future implant.

Glissan[4] first described specific principles of ankle arthrodesis. In 1949, he published his procedure describing 4 goals for fixation of ankle arthrodesis leading to higher fusion rates. First, he stressed the importance of removing all cartilage and tissue that would prevent intimate approximation of adjacent bony surfaces. The subsequent keys to union included a close-fitting construct for the fusion with optimal positioning of the fusion site.[4] In addition, maintenance of correction without interruption during the fusion period was pivotal for successful outcome.[4–6] AO technique, formally known as Arbeitsgemeinschaft für Osteosynthesefragen, expounded on Glissan's principles[4] of arthrodesis to produce fixation concepts currently adhered to today.

Over time, the principles of arthrodesis have remained largely unchanged; however, fixation modalities have progressed drastically. Initially fixation consisted of cadaveric allograft, ivory, fibular autograft, or suture and was followed by extended periods of immobilization. Despite adherence to strict non–weight bearing, materials and surgical techniques did not afford high union rates.[7]

At present, ankle arthrodesis uses a variety of fixation techniques, including internal screw fixation, external fixation, intramedullary nails, plates, and arthroscopic approaches (**Fig. 1**). When combined with correct surgical approach, each of these fixation techniques has resulted in high rates of fusion. In addition to changes in fixation techniques, which are discussed later, the incision approaches have also changed.

Indications

Ankle arthrodesis has numerous applications given advancements in surgical approaches and fixation techniques. The procedure remains at the forefront of treatment of advanced ankle arthritis. Ankle arthrosis and concomitant articular damage are often the result of previous trauma (**Fig. 2**). Injuries resulting in arthritis include crush injuries, comminuted fractures, and ankle instability with history of repetitive sprains.[8] Although posttraumatic arthritis is the primary indication for ankle arthrodesis,[5,6] the procedure can be used to treat congenital and neuromuscular disorders, infection, avascular necrosis of the talus, advanced posterior tibial tendon dysfunction, and Charcot neuroarthropathy, and serves as a salvage procedure for failed total ankle arthroplasty (**Fig. 3**).[5,9]

Contraindications

Contraindications for ankle arthrodesis are similar to those for other surgical interventions. Ankle arthrodesis for patients with multiple comorbidities who are medically unstable to undergo an elective procedure should be avoided until the patients are able to do so. In addition, local surgical site factors such as peripheral vascular disease and poor soft tissue quality from conditions such as lymphedema or venous disease should serve as deterrents from ankle arthrodesis.[5,8] Social factors such as tobacco use and excessive alcohol consumption, and ongoing psychological conditions must also be evaluated during risk/benefit analysis, because these conditions may produce unsatisfactory results.[10] Smoking is a relative contraindication, as shown in previous studies with increased nonunion rates in smokers compared with

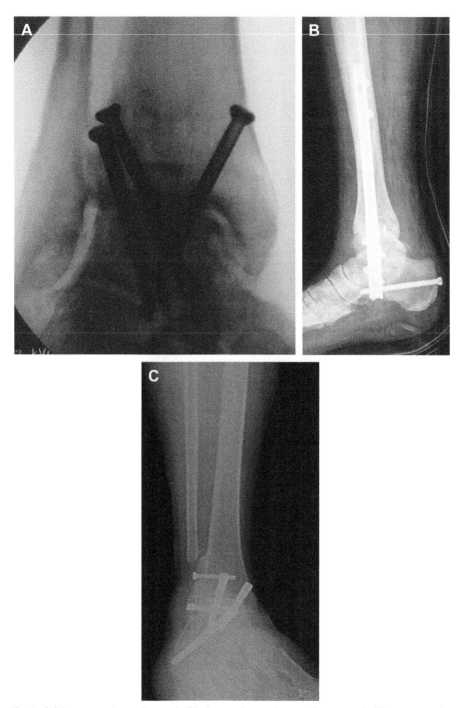

Fig. 1. (*A*) Postoperative radiograph: fibular sparing, arthroscopic approach. (*B*) Postoperative radiograph: intramedullary arthrodesis. (*C*) Traditional fibular-sacrificing ankle arthrodesis.

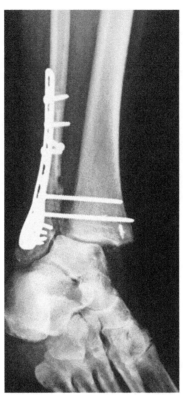

Fig. 2. A 54-year-old woman referred to clinic after poor reduction following ankle fracture dislocation.

nonsmokers.[10,11] In addition, nonunions have been noted to occur in up to one-third of patients using alcohol.[10]

PATIENT OVERVIEW: CLINICAL ASSESSMENT

During surgical consultation, patient history is of exceptional importance. Past trauma or injury leading to secondary ankle arthrosis should be highlighted; specifically past fractures, sprains, instability, and cartilaginous injuries. Approximately 50% of ankle arthritis is posttraumatic in origin.[6] It is important to note whether past trauma involved an open fracture because previous studies have shown that history of open fracture is a predilection for nonunion.[10]

A thorough past medical history should also be ascertained to determine the existence of gout, inflammatory arthritis, and avascular necrosis. Other systemic diseases affecting healing potential, such as diabetes mellitus, peripheral neuropathy, and vascular disease, must be addressed.[8] The presence of neuropathy or prior history of ulceration have proved to negatively affect bone healing.[12] Poorly controlled diabetic patients with hemoglobin A1c levels of 7% or greater are known to experience increased infectious and noninfectious complications in the postoperative period.[13] In addition, uncontrolled diabetics in another study were found to be at a 3-times greater risk of bone healing complications.[12] Other known risk factors of nonunion following arthrodesis are body mass index more than 30 and increased

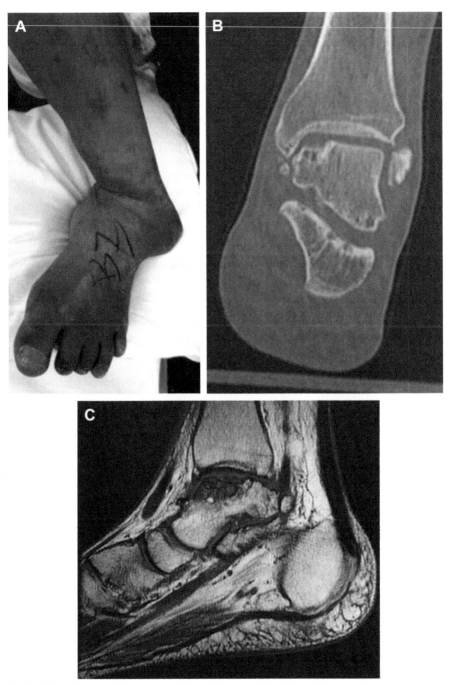

Fig. 3. (*A*) A 51-year-old woman with end-stage ankle deformity secondary to neuromuscular disorder. (*B*) Computed tomography (CT) image of severe talar collapse, secondary to trauma. (*C*) MRI talus showing significant talar disease.

age.[14] Special attention should be paid to medications, particularly to immunosuppressant medications, which have been recognized to negatively affect bone and wound healing.[15]

Physical examination should include evaluation of baseline neurovascular status as well as static and gait examination. When evaluating the lower extremity, areas of tenderness can elucidate various disorders aside from end-stage arthritis. Posteromedial pain could indicate dysfunction of the posterior tibial tendon. Subfibular discomfort could be a result of soft tissue or tendinous impingement. An additional method of differentiating ankle versus other joint or soft tissue involvement is a diagnostic local anesthetic injection. Complete relief following injection of the ankle joint eliminates adjacent joints as the source of pain, and is associated with better patient outcomes if ankle arthrodesis is performed.[6] During biomechanical examination, evaluation of rearfoot alignment as well as limitations in ankle dorsiflexion should be noted. Presence of excessive rearfoot varus, valgus, or equinus[16] should be thoroughly assessed in preoperative evaluation, because these conditions may require additional surgical procedures and affect potential nonunion rates.[17]

Weight-bearing radiographs of anteroposterior, lateral, and mortise views of the ankle should be obtained.[18] In addition to ankle views, a long calcaneal axial image and rearfoot alignment view should be ordered to evaluate the relationship of the calcaneus, subtalar joint, and the tibia.[16,18,19] Moreover, the center of rotation of angulation (CORA) must be evaluated on these images, because this point defines the apex of the deformity. At the ankle, CORA is best visualized at the lateral talar process on a lateral radiograph, which should align with the mid-diaphysial line of the tibia on lateral views.[20] The plantigrade angle between the tibia and the sole of the weight-bearing foot, measured perpendicular to the floor, should be 90°.[20] Advanced imaging studies such as computed tomography (CT) and MRI are reserved for cases requiring additional evaluation of osseous changes or soft tissue involvement.[16]

In addition, baseline analysis of vitamin D levels should be determined. Vitamin D levels of less than 30 ng/mL are known to impair healing. Recent studies have shown a prevalence of hypovitaminosis D.[21] Vitamin D is known to be a factor in fracture healing[22] and it could be extrapolated that correction of a deficiency before fusion is likely to be advantageous for the healing process.

Although the main goal of ankle arthrodesis is to provide a stable, plantigrade, and painless foot, concerns remain regarding stress placed on adjacent joints. Prior studies have shown that sagittal range of motion in the midfoot and hindfoot is unchanged after ankle arthrodesis compared with the unaffected contralateral limb.[23] Another recent study also found no significant differences in biomechanics following ankle fusion, possibly caused by compensation from the contralateral limb.[24] In contrast, development or progression of arthritis in adjacent joints is known to occur often, possibly necessitating an additional fusion in the future.[25] Zwipp and colleagues[26] showed the development or progression of arthritis in 35% of patients at the subtalar joint and in 18% of patients at the talonavicular joint. Increase in postarthrodesis arthritis may be caused by increased sagittal plane movement in the forefoot and increased transverse plane movements in both rearfoot and forefoot.[27]

Preoperative consultation must also include mentally preparing the patient for ankle arthrodesis and the required postoperative care. Patients should display understanding that they will be non–weight bearing for an extended period of time, at risk for complications, and may have continued limitation in function of their affected extremities. An in-depth discussion of postoperative plans, including possible entry to a rehabilitation facility and pain management regimen, should be highlighted as well.

SURGICAL TREATMENT OPTIONS
Technique

The technique for performing an open ankle arthrodesis has the same basics steps of any joint arthrodesis: incision, dissection preserving vital structures and maintaining vascularity, joint preparation, positioning, rigid fixation, and closure. When indicated, the use of arthrodesis-enhancing materials should be considered.

Incision Placement

Before planning incision placement, the surgeon must consider what the goals are for the patient. One initial question should be: after arthrodesis, will this patient ever be a candidate for a total ankle joint replacement (TAR)? For example, a patient who is too young or obese on initial examination may in several decades meet the criteria for a TAR simply by aging or losing weight. If this is a possibility or goal, then the transfibular approach with a fibular take-down should not be considered. In these cases, an anterior arthrotomy or miniarthrotomy approach would be preferred.

Another important consideration for incision placement is preexisting deformities in the operative limb. Significant varus or valgus eliminates either a miniarthrotomy approach or arthroscopic arthrodesis.[28] In the presence of deformity, the transfibular approach provides the best exposure for correction.[3] This approach, when combined with a medial ankle arthrotomy, has been a standard approach throughout the history of open ankle arthrodesis.

For the transfibular approach, the senior author prefers to position the patient on a beanbag in the lateral decubitus position with a thigh tourniquet. An incision is then created directly over the midline or slightly posterior to the midline of the distal one-third of the fibula (**Fig. 4**). It is carried inferiorly in a J-shaped fashion over the tip of the fibular malleolus. If a concomitant subtalar, calcaneocuboid, or a pantalar fusion is being performed, the J incision may be modified and carried anteriorly over the sinus tarsi and foot, ending at the base of the fourth metatarsal.

Dissection

When performing an isolated ankle arthrodesis, the incision is deepened and under-mining is not necessary until deeper layers are entered. Next, dissection is carried directly to the fibula and the periosteum is removed to expose the distal one-third of the fibula. Care must be taken to protect the sural nerve, perforating artery, and the peroneal tendons. A beveled osteotomy is created from superolateral to inferomedial, and can be created immediately above the ankle joint or, as the senior author prefers, taking several centimeters of the distal shaft that can be used as autogenous graft if needed later (**Fig. 5**).[29] The beveling of the osteotomy prevents irritation of the distal stump postoperatively. The fibula is then sharply removed by transecting all soft tissue attachments, including the collateral and syndesmotic ligaments, joint capsule, and interosseous membrane. A synostosis may exist between the fibula and tibia when severe degenerative changes have occurred as a result of previous injury or trauma. The synostosis may require removal with an osteotome or saw. One technical pearl for removing the fibula, with or without a synostosis, is using a sharp curved osteotome and passing it between the fibula and tibia to cut through the interosseous membrane and syndesmotic ligaments, and subsequently prying the fibula away from the ankle joint.

Once the fibula is removed, the ankle joint has complete exposure from anterior to posterior. If an in-situ fusion is being performed in the absence of varus/valgus deformity, minimal capsular dissection can be performed. However, if an end-to-end

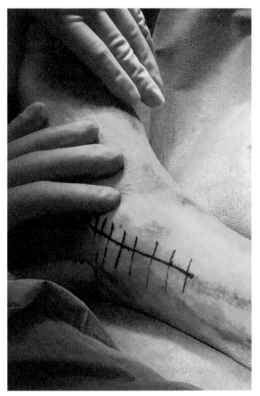

Fig. 4. Lateral incision for fibular-sacrificing ankle arthrodesis.

tabletop technique is to be used, the capsule and distal periosteum of the tibia is usually reflected both anteriorly and posteriorly from the joint using a Cobb-type elevator. Once the lateral dissection is completed, the leg can be externally rotated or the beanbag deflated to create a medial arthrotomy to expose the medial gutter and shoulder of the ankle.

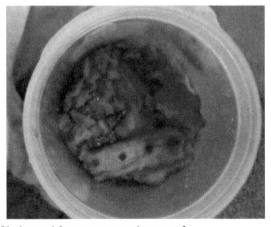

Fig. 5. Discarded fibula used for autogenous bone graft.

Joint Preparation

Once the joint surfaces have been exposed it is time for the joint preparation. If minimal deformity exists, the cartilage can simply be removed using various hand instruments such as curettes, ronguers, and osteotomes. Thickness of ankle cartilage ranges from 1.0 to 1.7 mm.[6] This task can be arduous, but it is essential to remove all of the cartilage from the joint surfaces. It is important to use the medial portal to remove the cartilage from the medial side of the joint. Avoid the temptation of using a bur to remove the cartilage because it may burn the underlying bone or create deformity by overzealous burring in certain areas.[5] In patients with osteoporosis, large pieces of bone or divots can easily be created using a bur.

For those patients requiring correction of varus or valgus, or when a table-top fusion (such as when using a lateral plate for fixation) is preferred, then the use of a saw is needed to create the appropriate wedge. The senior author prefers making a straight cut on the tibia and making the correction on the talus. When correcting for varus or valgus, the talus should be aligned 90° to the tibia while making the lateral to medial cut to ensure the proper position in both the sagittal and frontal planes. One potential pitfall when sawing from lateral to medial is that the surgeon can cut through or fracture the medial malleolus when removing the tibial cut. Some surgeons remove the medial gutter cartilage by hand first, and then use a saw to cut from anterior to posterior through the tibia. This method creates a breakaway point for the tibial cut. Others leave the saw blade in the anterior to posterior cut to avoid cutting the medial malleolus when cutting lateral to medial.[6] If these steps are performed properly, the cut should be of minimal height so as not to create a vertical fracture of the malleolus.

After removing all of the cartilage from the joint, the joint surfaces should be fenestrated to promote bleeding. Often in posttraumatic arthritis the subchondral plate is thick and requires using a small osteotomy to break through it, creating small chips (so-called fish scaling).

Positioning

Before fixation, the proper position for fusion should be achieved. It is the senior author's opinion that, although a nonunion can be a challenging reconstruction, a malunion can be even more challenging. The foot should be positioned 90° to the leg with 5° to 10° external rotation and slight heel valgus of 2°.[5,6,9,16,26,30] One potential pitfall is not adequately assessing any existing deformity proximal to the fusion site. Tibial varum, valgum, recurvatum, femoral/hip deformity, or existing limb length discrepancy may affect position or require correction either at the time of arthrodesis or before fusion.[9]

Fixation

Fixation of the open ankle arthrodesis may be achieved with multiple constructs. The use of large-diameter screws is a common technique and may be in the form of 2 screws, 2 screws with an onlay fibular bone graft, 3 screws, or a combination of screws with other forms of fixation. Screws can provide a rigid construct that provides compression and combats shearing forces, and is technically easy to perform. When using a 2-screw construct, they are typically crossed in 2 planes for enhanced stability. This technique should be accomplished in both the frontal and sagittal planes. When adding a third screw, it is usually placed from posterior to anterior, beginning in the tibia and ending in the anterior talar body or even the neck. This method can be technically challenging, especially when trying to avoid the previously placed screws. Despite the difficult placement of an additional screw, the tripod effect does help eliminate rotational forces and reduces micromotion at the fusion site[31] as well as providing additional compression.[32] Onlay fibular graft consisting of splitting the previously removed fibular shaft and removing the malleolus can accomplish the same benefits and also provides an opportunity for extra-articular arthrodesis (**Fig. 6**). One criticism of placing multiple large-diameter screws is that the screws potentially occupy a large portion of the arthrodesis site. For example, a tripod construct with 7.3-mm screws results in a 78% increase in screw area compared with two 6.5-mm screws, and uses 16% of the talar surface area to achieve arthrodesis.[33] However, when talar surface area was examined using anatomic bone models, an additional 6.5-mm or 7.0-mm screw did not significantly decrease bony availability for arthrodesis.[33]

Plates are an additional viable option for fixation. Given advancements in plate technology, they can provide compression in addition to neutralization. They are an excellent consideration in failed arthrodesis in which screws were previously used, because it is often challenging to find areas where screw placement could be successfully achieved in the reconstruction. A study by Doets and Zürcher[34] reported a 100% union rate in revisional arthrodesis for failed total ankle arthroplasty in patients in whom a plate was used for fixation.[34] In addition, screw fixation may lead to bony compromise if a graft is used to overcome a structural deficit following failed total ankle arthroplasty, making a plate the preferred fixation technique.[35]

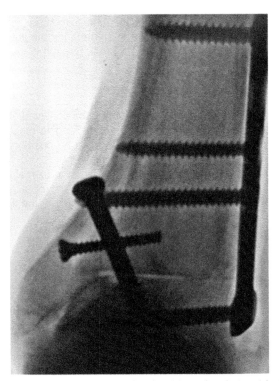

Fig. 6. Immediate postoperative radiograph of ankle arthrodesis with fibular-sacrificing procedure secondary to end-stage arthritis with frontal plane deformity from a prior ankle fracture.

External fixation may also serve a role, particularly in the Charcot ankle and revision. Some may argue that it is also a consideration in potentially noncompliant or obese patients who may weight bear postoperatively. Biomechanical evaluation of bone composites resulted in increased rigidity compared with cross screw construct, possibly reducing failure during early weight bearing postoperatively.[36] Intramedullary nails may also be used if performing a tibiotalar-calcaneal arthrodesis either primarily or for reconstruction. Staples may serve as a secondary point of fixation in certain cases but rarely should be used alone.

Anterior Approach to Ankle Arthrodesis

It has become increasingly popular with younger patients to perform a malleolar-sparing ankle arthrodesis to preserve the ability for conversion to an ankle replacement at a later date.

First, the anterior ankle joint line is identified in addition to the tibialis anterior (TA) and extensor halluces longus (EHL). Using the interval between the TA and EHL, a longitudinal incision is created, starting approximately 10 cm proximal to the ankle joint and 1 cm lateral to the tibial crest. The incision is carried distally to the talonavicular joint. Care should be taken to apply as little tension as possible on the skin margins to minimize risk of skin complications. The incision is deepened and dissection is continued without undermining. Next, the extensor retinaculum is exposed and the EHL course identified. As the retinaculum is transected, the retinaculum over the TA tendon is preserved to prevent bowstringing and subsequent stress on the anterior incision site. The EHL is retracted laterally and the TA medially. The deep neurovascular bundle is then retracted laterally. Next, an anterior capsulotomy is performed and reflected off the ankle joint in standard fashion to visualize the medial and lateral ankle gutters. Any anterior osteophytes can be removed at this time. At this point, adequate joint exposure has been achieved and it is time to proceed with joint preparation. Joint preparation and fixation principles are identical to the previously described technique for the transfibular approach.

Miniarthrotomy Ankle Arthrodesis

The TA is identified at the level of the ankle joint and a 2.5-cm incision is made medial to the tendon. The incision is deepened through the subcutaneous tissue with care taken to avoid the saphenous nerve and vein. The retinaculum is incised and the TA tendon retracted. In our experience, using a rongeur to remove any osteophytes or hypertrophied scar tissue can greatly enhance visualization and working space. A straight hemostat is driven through the incision and across the anterior joint to confirm the placement of the lateral incision. At this time, a second 2.5-cm incision is made lateral to the peroneus tertius tendon. Identical dissection is performed laterally as was performed medially, which allows complete visualization of the anterior joint and joint preparation can begin. Preparation and fixation principles are identical to those described in the transfibular approach.

Note that, with the arthrotomy approach, the posterior aspect of the joint often cannot be properly prepared. This inability makes proper joint preparation of 75% to 80% of the anterior joint of exceptional importance and vital to a successful outcome.

Orthobiologics

Orthobiologics can exist in many forms. Some of the more common forms are bone morphogenetic proteins, autogenous or allogenic bone graft, bone marrow, stem cells, various bone matrixes, and combinations thereof. Typically, these are used for patients at high risk of delayed union or nonunion.[37] These patients can be those who were discussed previously in this article who have comorbidities, medication or social habits that decrease healing potential. Patients with collagen vascular disease, diabetes mellitus, previous cancer, and bariatric surgery are the typical populations that may require supplementation to fixation in the form of an orthobiologic. A systematic review of foot and ankle arthrodesis procedures elucidated that application of graft, whether autograft or allograft, reduced the nonunion from 10% to approximately 4% when supplemental material was introduced.[38] Revisional arthrodesis patients and those with vitamin D deficiency may benefit from arthrodesis-enhancing materials, techniques, and orthobiologics as well. Bone stimulation in certain patients should also be considered.

POSTOPERATIVE CARE

Following surgery, the patient is placed in a compressive dressing with a posterior splint and is non–weight bearing. The patient is admitted for 1 to 2 days for postoperative pain management and observation. During outpatient follow-up, the patient is placed into a non–weight-bearing short leg cast for 6 to 8 additional weeks once the incisions are healed. If radiographs and clinical examination indicate signs of early arthrodesis, then the patient is transitioned to a fracture boot and progresses from partial to full weight bearing over the next month. After clinical and radiographic signs of union are noted, physical therapy and gradual progression to shoe gear occurs. Patients should be aware that recovery could be lengthy, because the average time to complete fusion in the ankle can be 26 weeks.[39] In the senior author's practice, the entire process takes a total of 4 to 6 months, with residual patient satisfaction issues (eg, edema, transition to shoes/activities) lasting up to a year.

COMPLICATIONS

The standard potential complications following lower extremity surgery, including but not limited to infection, wound issues, nerve entrapment, and deep vein thrombosis/pulmonary embolism, can occur following arthrodesis. However, ankle arthrodesis has additional concerns. Delayed union and nonunion have been reported at various rates. Recent literature has reported nonunion rates at 0% to 9% following open ankle arthrodesis.[17,40,41] As previously mentioned, multiple factors contribute to an individual's likelihood of developing such a complications, including comorbidities, social habits, fixation, and previous injury to the arthrodesis site.[10,11] Malunion and/or overshortening may lead to deleterious effects on the foot and knee, and may follow the closed kinetic chain to the hip and lower back. Shortening of the limb should be less than 1 cm if joint preparation for arthrodesis was properly performed.[5] In some cases hardware can cause pain, necessitating removal.

SUMMARY

Open ankle arthrodesis remains the gold standard treatment of advanced ankle arthritis. Physical examination is paramount to assess concomitant disorders that may need to be addressed before or during ankle arthrodesis. Although a variety of surgical approaches exist, adequate joint preparation, positioning, and fixation are fundamental to a successful procedure. As with any surgical procedure, complications may occur. However, these can be minimized by assessing risks preoperatively, patient compliance postoperatively, and appropriate approach and adjunctive procedures at the time of arthrodesis. Ankle arthrodesis can afford patients increased function with resolution of pain and previous symptoms.

REFERENCES

1. Albert E. Zur Resektion des Kniegelenkes. Wien Med Press 1879;20:705–8.
2. Charnley J. Compression arthrodesis of the ankle and shoulder. J Bone Joint Surg Br 1951;33:180–91.
3. Sung W, Greenhagen RM, Hobizal KB, et al. Technical guide: transfibular ankle arthrodesis with fibular-onlay strut graft. J Foot Ankle Surg 2010;49(6):566–70.
4. Glissan DJ. The indications for inducing fusion at the ankle joint by operation, with description of two successful techniques. ANZ J Surg 1949;19(1):64–71.
5. Deheer PA, Catoire SM, Taulman J, et al. Ankle arthrodesis. Clin Podiatr Med Surg 2012;29(4):509–27.
6. Bowers C, Catanzariti A, Mendicino R. Traditional ankle arthrodesis for the treatment of ankle arthritis. Clin Podiatr Med Surg 2009;26:259–71.
7. Campbell WC. Bone-block operation for drop-foot. J Bone Joint Surg 1929;27:317–24.
8. Boc SF, Norem ND. Ankle arthrodesis. Clin Podiatr Med Surg 2012;29(1):103–13.
9. Anderson RB, Saltzman CL, Coughlin MJ. Mann's surgery of the foot and ankle. 9th edition. Philadelphia: Saunders/Elsevier; 2014.
10. Perlman MH, Thordarson DB. Ankle fusion in a high risk population: an assessment of nonunion risk factors. Foot Ankle Int 1999;20(8):491–6.
11. Bender D, Jefferson-Keil T, Biglari B, et al. Cigarette smoking and its impact on fracture healing. Trauma 2013;16(1):18–22.
12. Shibuya N, Humphers JM, Fluhman BL, et al. Factors associated with nonunion, delayed union and malunion in foot and ankle surgery in diabetic patients. J Foot Ankle Surg 2013;52(2):207–11.
13. Myers TG, Lowery NJ, Frykberg RG, et al. Ankle and hindfoot fusions: comparison of outcomes in patients with and without diabetes. Foot Ankle Int 2012;33(1):20–8.
14. Thevendran G, Wang C, Pinney SJ, et al. Nonunion risk assessment in foot and ankle surgery: proposing a predictive risk assessment model. Foot Ankle Int 2015;36(8):901–7.
15. Grennan DM, Gray J, Loudon J, et al. Methotrexate and early postoperative complications in patients with rheumatoid arthritis undergoing elective orthopaedic surgery. Ann Rheum Dis 2001;60:214–7.
16. Grunfeld R, Aydogan U, Juliano P, et al. Ankle arthritis: diagnosis and conservative management. Med Clin North Am 2013;1(4):267–89.
17. Chalayon O, Wang B, Blankenhorn B, et al. Factors affecting the outcomes of uncomplicated primary open ankle arthrodesis. Foot Ankle Int 2015;36(10):1170–9.
18. Mendicino RW, Lamm BM, Catanzariti AR, et al. Realignment arthrodesis of the rearfoot and ankle. J Am Podiatr Med Assoc 2005;95(1):60–71.
19. Mendicino RW, Catanzariti AR, John S, et al. Long leg calcaneal axial and hindfoot alignment radiographic views for frontal plane assessment. J Am Podiatr Med Assoc 2008;98(1):75–8.
20. Lamm BM, Paley D. Deformity correction planning for hindfoot, ankle and lower limb. Clin Podiatr Med Surg 2004;21(3):305–26.
21. Michelson JD, Charlson MD. Vitamin D status in an elective orthopedic surgical population. Foot Ankle Int 2015;37(2):186–91.

22. Gorter EA, Hamdy NA, Appelman-Dijkstra NM, et al. The role of vitamin D in human fracture healing: a systematic review of the literature. Bone 2014;64:288–97.
23. van der Plaat LW, van Engelen SJ, Wajer QE, et al. Hind- and midfoot motion after ankle arthrodesis. Foot Ankle Int 2015;36(12):1430–7.
24. Fuentes-Sanz A, Moya-Angeler J, López-Oliva F, et al. Clinical outcome and gait analysis of ankle arthrodesis. Foot Ankle Int 2012;33(10):819–27.
25. Coester LM, Saltzman CL, Leupold J, et al. Long-term results following ankle arthrodesis for post-traumatic arthritis. J Bone Joint Surg Am 2001;83:219–28.
26. Zwipp H, Rammelt S, Endres T, et al. High union rates and function scores at midterm follow-up with ankle arthrodesis using a four screw technique. Clin Orthop Relat Res 2010;468(4):958–68.
27. Wu W-L, Su F-C, Cheng Y-M, et al. Gait analysis after ankle arthrodesis. Gait Posture 2000;11(1):54–61.
28. Nielsen KK, Linde F, Jensen NC. The outcome of arthroscopic and open surgery ankle arthrodesis. Foot Ankle Surg 2008;14(3):153–7.
29. Schuberth JM, Ruch JA, Hansen ST Jr. The tripod fixation technique for ankle arthrodesis. J Foot Ankle Surg 2009;48(1):93–6.
30. Buck P, Morrey BF, Chao EY. The optimum position of arthrodesis of the ankle: a gait study of the knee and ankle. J Bone Joint Surg Am 1987;69(7):1052–62.
31. Alonso-Vázquez A, Lauge-Pedersen H, Lidgren L, et al. Initial stability of ankle arthrodesis with three-screw fixation. A finite element analysis. Clin Biomech 2004;19(7):751–9.
32. Ogilvie-Harris DJ, Fitsialos D, Hedman TP. Arthrodesis of the ankle: a comparison of two-versus three-screw fixation in a crossed configuration. Clin Orthop Relat Res 1994;304:195–9.
33. Brodsky AR, Bohne WH, Huffard B, et al. An analysis of talar surface area occupied by screw fixation in ankle fusions. Foot Ankle Int 2006;27(1):53–5.
34. Doets HC, Zürcher AW. Salvage arthrodesis for failed total ankle arthroplasty. Acta Orthop 2010;81(1):142–7.
35. Espinosa N, Wirth SH, Jankauskas L. Ankle fusion after failed total ankle replacement. Tech Foot Ankle Surg 2010;9(4):199–204.
36. Hoover JR, Santrock RD, James WC. Ankle fusion stability: a biomechanical comparison of external versus internal fixation. Orthopedics 2011;34(4):272–7.
37. Bibbo C, Patel DV, Haskell MD. Recombinant bone morphogenetic protein-2 (rhBMP-2) in high-risk ankle and hindfoot fusions. Foot Ankle Int 2009;30(7):597–603.
38. Lareau CR, Deren ME, Fantry A, et al. Does autogenous bone graft work A logistic regression analysis of data from 159 papers in the foot and ankle literature. Foot Ankle Surg 2015;21(3):150–9.
39. Mirmiran R, Wilde B, Nielsen M. Retrospective analysis of the rate and interval to union for joint arthrodesis of the foot and ankle. J Foot Ankle Surg 2015;53(4):420–5.
40. Lee H-J, Min W-K, Kim J-S, et al. Transfibular ankle arthrodesis using burring, curettage, multiple drilling and fixation with two retrograde screws through a single lateral incision. J Orthop Surg 2016;24(1):101–5.
41. Akra GA, Middleton A, Adedapo AO, et al. Outcome of ankle arthrodesis using a transfibular approach. J Foot Ankle Surg 2010;49(6):508–12.

Arthroscopic Ankle Arthrodesis: An Update

Jason A. Piraino, DPM, MS[a], Michael S. Lee, DPM, MS[b],*

KEYWORDS

• Ankle • Arthrodesis • Arthroscopy • Fusion • Arthritis

KEY POINTS

- Arthroscopic ankle arthrodesis provides the foot and ankle surgeon with an alternative to traditional open techniques.
- Arthroscopic ankle arthrodesis has demonstrated faster rates of union, fewer complications, reduced postoperative pain, and shorter hospital stays.
- Adherence to sound surgical techniques, particularly with regard to joint preparation, is critical for success.
- Comorbidities such as increased body mass index, history of smoking, malalignment, and posttraumatic arthritis, should be considered carefully when contemplating arthroscopic ankle arthrodesis.
- Although total ankle replacement continues to grow in popularity, arthroscopic ankle arthrodesis remains a viable alternative for management of the end-stage arthritic ankle.

Ankle arthrodesis remains the gold standard for the treatment of end-stage ankle arthritis despite the increasing popularity and utilization of total ankle replacement.[1,2] High complication rates have been noted with total ankle replacement procedures at both intermediate and long-term follow-up.[3,4] Historically, open techniques have been used for ankle arthrodesis. There have been numerous approaches described including transfibular, anterior, medial, and miniarthrotomy.[5–19] Inherent disadvantages to these open techniques include postoperative pain, delayed union or nonunion, wound complications, shortening of the operative extremity, prolonged healing times, and prolonged hospital stays.[20–22]

Arthroscopic ankle arthrodesis provides the foot and ankle surgeon with an alternative to the traditional open techniques. Compared with open techniques, arthroscopic

This is an updated version of an article that originally appeared in *Clinics in Podiatric Medicine and Surgery*, Volume 26, Issue 2.

[a] Foot and Ankle Surgery, Podiatric Medicine and Surgery Residency, Department of Orthopaedics and Rehabilitation, University of Florida College of Medicine-Jacksonville, 655 West 8th Street, Jacksonville, FL 32209, USA; [b] Foot and Ankle Surgery, Capital Orthopaedics and Sports Medicine, PC, 12499 University Avenue, Suite 210, Clive, IA 50325, USA
* Corresponding author.
E-mail address: mlee@dsmcapitalortho.com

Clin Podiatr Med Surg 34 (2017) 503–514
http://dx.doi.org/10.1016/j.cpm.2017.05.007
0891-8422/17/© 2017 Elsevier Inc. All rights reserved.

ankle arthrodesis has demonstrated faster union rates, fewer complications, reduced postoperative pain, and shorter hospital stays.[5,22–31] Although once considered technically demanding, advancements in techniques and instrumentation have shortened the learning curve once encountered with the arthroscopic technique.

Schneider[32] first reported arthroscopic ankle arthrodesis in 1983 and reported faster time to union, earlier mobilization, and reduced patient morbidity. More recent studies have demonstrated similar results with faster union rates, fewer complications, and shorter hospital stays with union rates comparable to more recent open techniques.[5,23–25,31] This article explores the indications, techniques, and complications associated with arthroscopic ankle arthrodesis.

INDICATIONS AND CONTRAINDICATIONS

Arthroscopic ankle arthrodesis may be indicated in patients with end-stage arthritis owing to a variety of etiologies, including rheumatoid arthritis, posttraumatic arthritis, arthrogryphosis, septic arthritis, inflammatory arthritis, avascular necrosis of the talus, idiopathic osteoarthritis, and chronic ankle instability. The most frequently encountered etiology remains posttraumatic arthritis, however.[23]

The primary indication for ankle arthrodesis is persistent pain that has not responded to conservative treatments including analgesics, nonsteroidal antiinflammatory drugs, corticosteroid injections, and orthoses or bracing.[5,24,30] Although not currently approved by the US Food and Drug Administration for the ankle joint, hyaluronase injections may also be considered before proceeding with arthrodesis or replacement.

Limitations of arthroscopic ankle arthrodesis are typically related to deformity or malalignment about the ankle joint. Various studies have indicated that malalignment greater than 10° to 15° will make reduction of the ankle joint and deformity difficult.[25,33] Ferkel and Hewitt[29] indicated that patients with significant ankle deformity, either significant varus or valgus, are better suited for an open technique and those that require arthrodesis in situ are better suited for the arthroscopic technique. Tang and colleagues[34] stated that arthroscopy should not be advised when a large ankle deformity is present. A study done in 2007 by Gougoulias and colleagues[28] showed that patients with marked deformity of greater than 10° to 15° of varus or valgus can be treated effectively using arthroscopy, depending on surgeon experience.

In addition to significant malalignment, Collman and colleagues[24] noted that contraindications of arthroscopic ankle arthrodesis include excessive bone loss, neuropathic joints, active infections, and poor bone stock. Avascular necrosis of the talus may also be a contraindication.

SURGICAL TECHNIQUE

Arthroscopic ankle arthrodesis is performed under general or spinal anesthesia. A thigh tourniquet is typically used for hemostasis and the leg is prepped to the tibial tuberosity. A bump under the ipsilateral hip is used to slightly internally rotate the leg.

Standard anteromedial and anterolateral portals are used. A 2.7-mm, 30° arthroscope is introduced into the ankle joint. The authors prefer to use large joint power shavers and burrs while using a 2.7-mm arthroscope rather than the 4.0 mm arthroscope. Arthroscopic instrumentation such as picks, osteotomes, and awls may also be helpful in tight areas. This allows access into the tibiotalar space to view the posterior half of the talar dome. A noninvasive ankle distractor is applied to the ankle to allow for complete visualization from anterior to posterior, as well as both the medial and lateral gutters (**Fig. 1**).

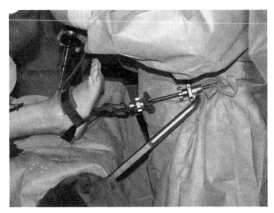

Fig. 1. Noninvasive ankle distracter being used for joint visualization. (*From* Lee MS, Millward DM. Arthroscopic ankle arthrodesis. Clin Podiatr Med Surg 2009;26(2):273–82; with permission.)

A 4.0-mm full radius incisor blade is used to aggressively debride the anterior joint of any hypertrophic synovium, fibrosis, or loose bodies. In some cases, aggressive resection of anterior tibiotalar osteophytes is required for proper joint visualization. A curette is used to aggressively remove any remaining articular cartilage (**Fig. 2**). A grasping forceps or resector may be used to remove the loose cartilage fragments, which typically collect in the posterior recess of the joint (**Fig. 3**). A 4.0-mm full radius burr or 4.5-mm acromion burr is then used to resect the subchondral plate (**Fig. 4**). A curved osteotome is then used to fish scale the subchondral plates of both the tibia and talus (**Fig. 5**). Ideally, healthy bleeding bone will be visualized throughout the tibiotalar articulation (**Fig. 6**). The joint is then irrigated and all loose bodies or fragments are evacuated.

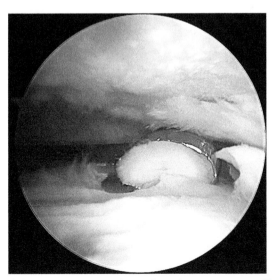

Fig. 2. Curettage of the remaining articular surface. (*From* Lee MS, Millward DM. Arthroscopic ankle arthrodesis. Clin Podiatr Med Surg 2009;26(2):273–82; with permission.)

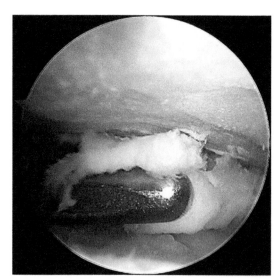

Fig. 3. Removal of the cartilage fragments after aggressive curettage. (*From* Lee MS, Millward DM. Arthroscopic ankle arthrodesis. Clin Podiatr Med Surg 2009;26(2):273–82; with permission.)

All arthroscopic instrumentation is then removed from the ankle joint. Platelet-rich plasma or other bone graft substitutes may then be inserted into the ankle joint at the surgeon's discretion. At this point, the noninvasive distractor may be removed from the foot. Proper bony apposition is confirmed using fluoroscopy. Care must be taken to confirm proper positioning clinically and radiographically. It is of vital importance to obtain multiple views to ensure appropriate positioning. Often, it is best to temporarily hold position with Steinman pins or large threaded K-wires.

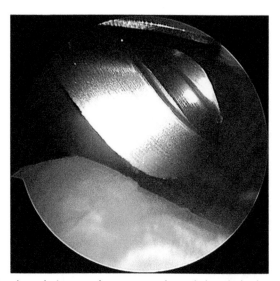

Fig. 4. Full radius burr being used to resect the subchondral plate. (*From* Lee MS, Millward DM. Arthroscopic ankle arthrodesis. Clin Podiatr Med Surg 2009;26(2):273–82; with permission.)

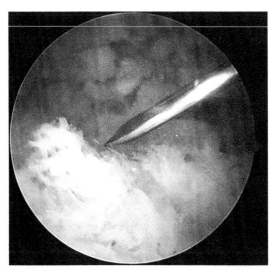

Fig. 5. Fish scaling the talus with a curved osteotome in preparation for arthrodesis. (*From* Lee MS, Millward DM. Arthroscopic ankle arthrodesis. Clin Podiatr Med Surg 2009;26(2):273–82; with permission.)

Fixation is achieved with 2 or 3 large diameter cannulated screws. Typically, 2 cannulated screws are stacked from the medial tibia into the talus with one directed slightly anterior to the other and a third screw is passed laterally through the fibula, across the syndesmosis into the distal tibia then across the joint into the medial talar body (**Fig. 7**).

The portals and stab incisions for screw placement are closed with simple sutures. The extremity is placed in a controlled ankle motion (CAM) boot. In most cases, the patient is discharged to home the day of surgery. Sutures are removed at 1 week

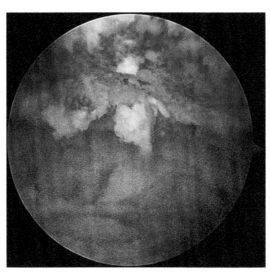

Fig. 6. Joint surfaces after preparation for arthrodesis. (*From* Lee MS, Millward DM. Arthroscopic ankle arthrodesis. Clin Podiatr Med Surg 2009;26(2):273–82; with permission.)

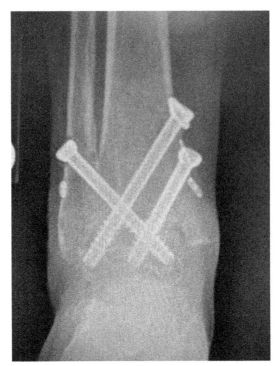

Fig. 7. Typical fixation after arthroscopic ankle arthrodesis.

postoperatively and the patient is placed in a below-the-knee cast, or may be maintained in the CAM walker. Strict adherence to non–weight bearing is followed for 6 to 7 weeks. Weight bearing is then advanced based on radiographic healing and clinical symptoms in a CAM boot (**Fig. 8**). Typically, at approximately 10 weeks postoperatively, the patient is placed in a rocker-bottom sole shoe and ankle-foot orthoses, and activities are advanced as tolerated. The ankle-foot orthoses is continued for up to an additional 3 months and the rocker-bottom sole is continued according to the patient's preference after 6 months.

DISCUSSION

Arthroscopic ankle arthrodesis has been well-studied and demonstrated favorable postoperative outcomes.[22–31] Advantages include decreased time to union, diminished postoperative pain, comparable union rates, shorter hospital stays, and earlier patient mobilization.[22–31,35–38] Preservation of the bony contour and the large amount of cancellous bony contact allows for significant stability and rigid internal fixation.[24,38] This is contradictory to the traditional open techniques, which have often implemented planal resection decreasing bony contact and decreasing inherent stability. Additionally, "flat topping" the talus and tibia makes proper positioning of the foot in the sagittal plane significantly more difficult, as precise bone cuts are required. O'Brien and colleagues[22] showed there was greater variability of ankle positions in patients that received the open ankle fusion compared with the arthroscopic technique.

Stetson and Ferkel[33] recommended an open technique in ankles that have malrotation or anterior-posterior translation of the tibiotalar joint. They also believed ankles

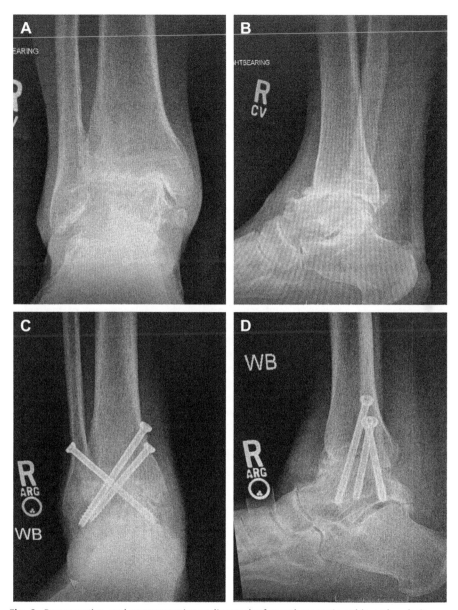

Fig. 8. Preoperative and postoperative radiographs for arthroscopic ankle arthrodesis.

that had a deformity of greater than 15° of varus or valgus should be treated with an open technique.[33] Gougoulias and colleagues,[28] however, achieved successful arthroscopic ankle arthrodeses on ankle deformities of 15° to 45° of varus or valgus. They point out that, although they were able to successfully fuse ankles with marked deformity, there is a significant learning curve associated with the procedure.[28] Another recent study also suggests that it may be possible to fuse ankles with deformities of 25° or greater arthroscopically.[25] The authors have found that malalignment of up to 15° is acceptable for arthroscopic arthrodesis. In some cases, particularly in severe valgus malalignment of the ankle, the joint may be reducible clinically. In these cases, arthroscopic ankle arthrodesis is possible but preoperative planning should include the possibility of converting to a miniarthrotomy.

Union may be described in 2 different ways: clinical union and radiographic union. Clinical union is described as having a stable, painless ankle joint. Radiographic union is defined as having bridging trabeculae between the tibia and the talus.[28,39]

Interestingly, nonunion rates between arthroscopic ankle arthrodesis and open techniques are similar. Collman and colleagues[24] reported a 93% clinical fusion rate and a 74% radiographic union rate, indicating a subset of arthroscopic ankle arthrodesis cases that have clinical union rate of 87.2%. Winson and colleagues[25] reported a nonunion rate of 7.6% in their review of 118 arthroscopic ankle fusions. Similar union rates in other studies have been reported with a range from 73% to 100%.[5,19,22,29–31,35,37,40–42]

Studies demonstrating union rates correlated to patient comorbidities have been limited primarily to rheumatoid arthritis.[41,43,44] Other variables such as history of smoking, arthritis etiology, effects of bone graft substitutes, body mass index, and preexisting deformity have not been extensively studied with regards to arthroscopic ankle arthrodesis. In 1 study, 4 of 5 patients reported nonunions in patients with posttraumatic arthritis.[24] The higher concentration of sclerotic bone adjacent to the subchondral plate may contribute to this increased incidence of nonunion, reinforcing the importance of aggressive joint resection.[31,35,43,45] Malalignment of the ankle may also predispose to nonunion of the arthroscopic ankle arthrodesis.[24]

Cigarette smoking and its negative effects on both soft tissue and bone healing has been well-documented (**Fig. 9**).[46–51] The role of nicotine in ankle arthrodesis nonunions has also been well-documented, and may present a relative risk of nonunion 4 times that seen in nonsmokers.[20,52] Collman and colleagues[24] did not see this same trend in their series of arthroscopic ankle fusions and theorized that the ill-effects of smoking are countered by the minimally invasive approach.

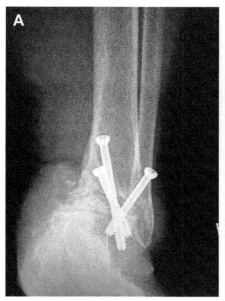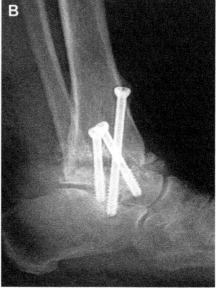

Fig. 9. Nonunion in a smoker.

A clear advantage to the use of arthroscopic arthrodesis over open techniques is the time to fusion is reduced. Open ankle fusions have a reported average fusion time of approximately 14 weeks.[35,36] In a study of 39 arthroscopic arthrodeses, Collman and colleagues[24] reported an average fusion time of 47 days, whereas Glick and colleagues[37] noted a 9-week average fusion time in 34 ankles. Other studies have noted time to fusion for arthroscopic ankle arthrodesis from 8.9 to 12.0 weeks.[5,25,31] One theory to support the decreased fusion time is that the arthroscopic technique does not disrupt the periarticular blood supply facilitating healing.[31,35,37,43]

O'Brien and associates[22] demonstrated that the tourniquet time, blood loss, and hospitalization times were all decreased using arthroscopy. Patients who underwent arthroscopic arthrodesis had hospital stays of 1.6 days, versus the open techniques that averaged 3.4 days in the hospital.[22] Use of the arthroscopic technique may greatly reduce the postoperative hospitalization period. Ogilvie-Harris and colleagues[30] reported an average discharge from the hospital of 1 day. Dent and colleagues[27] also reports an average stay of less than 2 days. Zvijac and colleagues[31] reported an average hospitalization of 3 days for those who had an open procedure as compared with 1 day for those who received an arthroscopic arthrodesis.[29] They noted pain levels where much less than expected in the arthroscopic group leading them to perform arthroscopic ankle arthrodesis on an outpatient basis. In yet another study, arthroscopic fusion compared with open techniques demonstrated significant cost savings.[53] Cameron and Ulrich[5] also reported doing arthroscopic ankle arthrodesis as an outpatient procedure. In another study of 39 patients, only 3 were not discharged the day of the procedure.[24]

Arthroscopic ankle arthrodesis has demonstrated reduced pain postoperatively as well as a shorter reliance on pain medication.[27,30,31] The authors have also noted a significant decrease in postoperative pain with the arthroscopic technique. It is now common practice for arthroscopic ankle arthrodeses to be performed in outpatient surgery centers and generally the decision to admit a patient postoperatively is based on comorbid deformities and not postoperative pain concerns.

Other advantages of arthroscopic arthrodesis include decreased blood loss, decreased disruption of the soft tissue structures about the ankle, and diminished risk of thrombosis owing to shorter immobilization times. There is also minimal loss of length of the lower limb, as well as minimal clinical deformity or shape changes to the ankle,[27] which can be quite beneficial if the patient ever is to be converted to total ankle joint replacement.

Arthroscopic ankle arthrodesis may be preferred to an open technique in at-risk patients.[24] The earlier mobilization owing to a shorter time to union is beneficial in patients with rheumatoid arthritis, advanced age, diabetes, and other autoimmune diseases.[35,42] The senior author has used the arthroscopic technique in these at-risk patients with great success, but cautions its use in patients with peripheral neuropathy.

SUMMARY

Arthroscopic ankle arthrodesis provides the foot and ankle surgeon with an alternative to traditional open techniques. Advancements in arthroscopic techniques and instrumentation have made the procedure easier to perform. Arthroscopic ankle arthrodesis has demonstrated faster rates of union, decreased complications, reduced postoperative pain, and shorter durations of hospital stay.[5,22–31] Adherence to sound surgical techniques, particularly with regard to joint preparation is critical for success. Comorbidities such as increased body mass index, history of smoking, malalignment, and posttraumatic arthritis should be carefully considered when contemplating arthro-scopic ankle arthrodesis. Although total ankle replacement continues to grow in popularity, arthroscopic ankle arthrodesis remains a viable alternative for management of the end-stage arthritic ankle.

REFERENCES

1. Coester LM, Saltman CL, Leapold J, et al. Long-term results following ankle arthrodesis for post-traumatic arthritis. J Bone Joint Surg Am 2001;83:219–28.
2. Buck P, Morrey BF, Chao EY. The optimum position of arthrodesis of the ankle. A gait study of the knee and ankle. J Bone Joint Surg Am 1987;69:1052–62.
3. Kwon DG, Chung CY, Park MS, et al. Arthroplasty versus arthrodesis for end-stage ankle arthritis: decision analysis using Markov model. Int Orthop 2011; 35:1647–53.
4. Daniels TR, Younger AS, Penner M, et al. Intermediate-term results of total ankle replacement and ankle arthrodesis: a COFAS multicenter study. J Bone Joint Surg Am 2014;96:135–42.
5. Cameron SE, Ullrich P. Arthroscopic arthrodesis of the ankle joint. Arthroscopy 2000;16:21–6.
6. Cheng YM, Chen SK, Chen JC, et al. Revision of ankle arthrodesis. Foot Ankle Int 2003;24:321–5.
7. Colgrove RC, Bruffey JD. Ankle arthrodesis: combined internal-external fixation. Foot Ankle Int 2001;22:92–7.
8. Adams JC. Arthrodesis of the ankle joint; experiences with transfibular approach. J Bone Joint Surg Br 1948;30B(3):506–11.
9. Frankel JP, Bacardi BE. Chevron ankle arthrodesis with bone grafting and internal fixation. J Foot Surg 1986;25:234–40.
10. Anderson R. Concentric arthrodesis of the ankle joint: a transmalleolar approach. J Bone Joint Surg 1945;27:37–48.
11. Baciu CC. A simple technique for arthrodesis of the ankle. J Bone Joint Surg 1986;68(2):266–7.
12. Campbell P. Arthrodesis of the ankle with modified distraction-compression and bone-grafting. J Bone Joint Surg Am 1990;72:552–6.
13. Campbell CJ, Rinehart WT, Kalenak A. Arthrodesis of the ankle: deep autogenous inlay grafts with maximum cancellous bone apposition. J Bone Joint Surg Am 1974;56:63–70.
14. Vogler HW. Ankle fusion: techniques and complications. J Foot Surg 1991;30: 80–4.
15. Thordarson DB, Markolf KL, Cracchiolo A. Arthrodesis of the ankle with cancellous-bone screws and fibular strut graft. Biomechanical analysis. J Bone Joint Surg Am 1990;72:1359–63.
16. Mauerer RC, Cimino WR, Cox CV, et al. Transarticular cross-screw fixation; a technique of ankle arthrodesis. Clin Orthop Relat Res 1991;(268):56–69.
17. Morgan CD, Henke JA, Bailey RW, et al. Long-term results of tibiotalar arthrodesis. J Bone Joint Surg Am 1985;67:546–50.
18. Mears DC, Gordon RG, Kann SE, et al. Ankle arthrodesis with an anterior tension plate. Clin Orthop 1991;268:70–7.
19. Paremain GD, Miller SD, Myerson MS. Ankle arthrodesis: results after the miniar-throtomy technique. Foot Ankle Int 1996;17:247–51.
20. Frey C, Halikus NM, Vu-Rose T, et al. A review of ankle arthrodesis: predisposing factors to nonunion. Foot Ankle Int 1994;15(11):581–4.

21. Morrey BF, Wiedeman GP Jr. Complications and long-term results of ankle arthrodeses following trauma. J Bone Joint Surg Am 1980;62(5):777–84.

22. O'Brien TS, Hart TS, Shereff MJ, et al. Open versus arthroscopic ankle arthrodesis: a comparative study. Foot Ankle Int 1999;20(6):368–74.

23. Stone JW. Arthroscopic ankle arthrodesis. Foot Ankle Clin 2006;11(2):361–8.

24. Collman DR, Kaas MH, Schuberth JM. Arthroscopic ankle arthrodesis: factors influencing union in 39 consecutive patients. Foot Ankle Int 2006;27:1079–85.

25. Winson IG, Robinson DE, Allen PE. Arthroscopic ankle arthrodesis. J Bone Joint Surg Br 2005;87(3):343–7.

26. Kats J, van Kampen A, de Waal-Malefijt MC. Improvement in technique for arthroscopic ankle fusion: results in 15 patients. Knee Surg Sports Traumatol Arthrosc 2003;11(1):46–9.

27. Dent CM, Patil M, Fairclough JA. Arthroscopic ankle arthrodesis. J Bone Joint Surg Br 1993;75(5):830–2.

28. Gougoulias NE, Agathangelidis FG, Parsons SW. Arthroscopic ankle arthrodesis. Foot Ankle Int 2007;28(6):695–706.

29. Ferkel RD, Hewitt M. Long-term results of arthroscopic ankle arthrodesis. Foot Ankle Int 2005;26(4):275–80.

30. Ogilvie-Harris DJ, Lieberman I, Fitsialos D. Arthroscopically assisted arthrodesis for osteoarthrotic ankles. J Bone Joint Surg Am 1993;75(8):1167–74.

31. Zvijac JE, Lemak L, Schurhoff MR, et al. Analysis of arthroscopically assisted ankle arthrodesis. Arthroscopy 2002;18(1):70–5.

32. Schneider D. Arthroscopic ankle fusion. Arthroscopic Video J 1983;3.

33. Stetson WB, Ferkel RD. Ankle arthroscopy: II. Indications and results. J Am Acad Orthop Surg 1996;4(1):24–34.

34. Tang KL, Li QH, Chen GX, et al. Arthroscopically assisted ankle fusion in patients with end-stage tuberculosis. Arthroscopy 2007;23(9):919–22.

35. Myerson MS, Quill G. Ankle arthrodesis. A comparison of an arthroscopic and an open method of treatment. Clin Orthop Relat Res 1991;(268):84–95.

36. Mann RA, Van Manen JW, Wapner K, et al. Ankle fusion. Clin Orthop Relat Res 1991;28:49–55.

37. Glick JM, Morgan CD, Myerson MS, et al. Ankle arthrodesis using an arthroscopic method: long-term follow-up of 34 cases. Arthroscopy 1996;12(4):428–34.

38. Jay RM. A new concept of ankle arthrodesis via arthroscopic technique. Clin Podiatr Med Surg 2000;17(1):147–57.

39. Monroe MT, Beals TC, Manoli A 2nd. Clinical outcome of arthrodesis of the ankle using rigid internal fixation with cancellous screws. Foot Ankle Int 1999;20(4):227–31.

40. Crosby LA, Yee TC, Formanek TS, et al. Complications following arthroscopic ankle arthrodesis. Foot Ankle Int 1996;17:340–2.

41. Corso SJ, Zimmer TJ. Technique and clinical evaluation of arthroscopic ankle arthrodesis. Arthroscopy 1995;11:585–90.

42. Jerosch J, Steinbeck J, Schroder M, et al. Arthroscopically assisted arthrodesis of the ankle joint. Arch Orthop Trauma Surg 1996;115:182–9.

43. DeVriese L, Dereymaeker G, Fabry G. Arthroscopic ankle arthrodesis preliminary report. Acta Orthop Belg 1994;60:389–92.

44. Turan I, Wredmark T, Fellander-Tsai L. Arthroscopic ankle arthrodesis in rheumatoid arthritis. Clin Orthop 1995;320:110–4.

45. Blair HC. Comminuted fractures and fracture-dislocations of the body of the astragalus: operative treatment. Am J Surg 1943;59:37–43.

46. Brown CW, Orme TJ, Richardson HD. The rate of pseudoarthrosis (surgical nonunion) in patients who are smokers and patients who are nonsmokers; a comparison study. Spine 1986;11:942–3.
47. Glasman SD, Anagnost SC, Parker A, et al. The effect of cigarette smoking and smoking cessation on spinal fusion. Spine 2000;25:2608–15.
48. Haverstock BD, Mandracchia VJ. Cigarette smoking and bone healing: implication in foot and ankle surgery. J Foot Ankle Surg 1998;37:69–74.
49. Ishikawa SN, Murphy GA, Richardson EG. The effect of cigarette smoking on hindfoot fusions. Foot Ankle Int 2002;23:996–8.
50. Nolan J, Jenkins RA, Kurihara K, et al. The acute effects of cigarette smoke exposure on experimental skin flaps. Plast Reconstr Surg 1985;75:544–51.
51. Sherwin MA, Gastwirth CM. Detrimental effects of cigarette smoking on lower extremity wound healing. J Foot Surg 1990;29:84–7.
52. Cobb TK, Gabrielsen TA, Campbell DC 2nd, et al. Cigarette smoking and nonunion after ankle arthrodesis. Foot Ankle 1994;15:64–7.
53. Petersen KS, Lee MS, Buddecke DE. Arthroscopic versus open ankle arthrodesis: a retrospective cost analysis. J Foot Ankle Surg 2010;49:242–7.

Current Concepts Regarding Total Ankle Replacement as a Viable Treatment Option for Advanced Ankle Arthritis: What You Need to Know

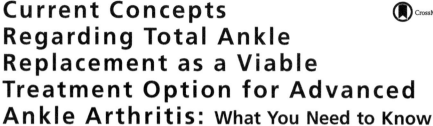

Christopher L. Reeves, DPM, FACFAS[a,b,*],
Amber M. Shane, DPM, FACFAS[b,c], Ryan Vazales, DPM[d]

KEYWORDS

- Ankle arthritis • Degenerative joint disease • Total ankle replacement
- Post traumatic ankle arthritis • Ankle arthroplasty

KEY POINTS

- The goal of any total ankle replacement (TAR) surgery is to improve function and decrease pain.
- Preoperative planning, including careful patient selection and exhaustive discussions with the patient regarding every aspect of the surgical treatment plan that includes possible complications and patient expectations regarding end results, is paramount to successful outcomes.
- Not all patients with end-stage ankle arthritis are candidates for a TAR procedure.
- Survivorship of TAR remains controversial; however, the newer generation, less constrained models are continuing to show improvement in reliability and functionality.
- TAR should no longer be considered a "fringe" or inferior procedure to ankle fusion but rather a viable alternative in the right patient population.

Financial Disclosure: The authors have nothing to disclose as it relates to the content of this article.
Conflict of Interest: Nothing to report.
[a] Orlando Foot and Ankle Clinic, 2111 Glenwood Drive, Suite 104, Winter Park, FL 32792, USA;
[b] Podiatric Surgical Residency Program, Department of Podiatric Surgery, Florida Hospital East Orlando, 7727 Lake Underhill Road, Orlando, FL 32828, USA; [c] Orlando Foot and Ankle Clinic, 250 North Alafaya Trail, Suite 115, Orlando, FL 32825, USA; [d] Residency Training Program, Podiatric Medicine and Surgery, Florida Hospital East Orlando, 7727 Lake Underhill Road, Orlando, FL 32828, USA
* Corresponding author. Orlando Foot and Ankle Clinic, 2111 Glenwood Drive, Suite 104, Winter Park, FL 32792.
E-mail address: docreeves1@yahoo.com

INTRODUCTION

End-stage ankle arthritis can be an extremely debilitating pathology affecting a patient's ability to carry out activities of daily life when severe. Multiple mechanisms of action associated with the underlying cause of ankle arthritis exist, including but not limited to degenerative joint disease, posttraumatic changes, abnormal biomechanics, and ankle instability (**Fig. 1**). Traditionally, ankle arthrodesis has been the gold standard for surgical correction of ankle arthritis when conservative methods have failed. However, total ankle replacement (TAR), has only recently been accepted as a mainstream surgical option for end-stage ankle arthritis as improvement in postsurgical outcomes have been recognized. Newer generation devices have done a better job of incorporating ankle joint biomechanical principles in their less constrained designs, which has led to better surgical outcomes.

Much of the current literature suggests that TAR is no longer an inferior or fringe treatment for advanced ankle arthritis compared with ankle fusion, but rather a viable option for recalcitrant arthritic ankle pathology in the correct patient population.[1] In this article, current concepts associated with successful outcomes for TAR are discussed, with an emphasis on ankle joint anatomy and biomechanics, preoperative planning and patient selection, understanding pathomechanics (center of rotational angulation [CORA]) and soft tissue balancing, as well as the surgeon's learning curve.

ANKLE JOINT ANATOMY AND BIOMECHANICS

Much of the discussion regarding ankle joint anatomy and biomechanics as it relates to TAR center around the notion of triplanar movement and coupled motion, which has explained the failures in first-generation and second-generation total ankle devices. The earlier generation device's inability to account for triplanar rotational components of the tibiotalar joint, as well as relying on more constrained constructs, contributed to poor outcomes and an idea of inferiority to the gold standard ankle arthrodesis. However, newer models of TAR seem to have recognized this previous flaw, and adjustments have been made to accommodate biomechanical function.

The tibiotalar joint is stabilized by 2 ligamentous complexes. Laterally, the joint houses 3 ligamentous structures, including the anteroinferior tibiofibular ligament, the postero-inferior tibiofibular ligament, and the interosseous tibiofibular ligament, which is a continuation of the interosseous membrane. This structure, known as the lateral collateral ligament complex of the ankle, acts to allow the distal tibia and fibula to function as one unit when adapting to changes in ground reactive forces being applied. Medially, the ankle joint is stabilized by the deltoid ligament, with both

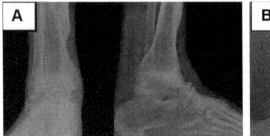 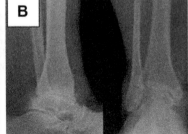

Fig. 1. Anteroposterior and lateral view of posttraumatic degenerative joint disease of the ankle (*A*). Anteroposterior and lateral views of primary osteoarthritis to the ankle (*B*).

superficial and deep attachments known as the medial collateral ligament complex of the ankle. The inferior lateral ligament complex is composed of the anterior talofibular ligament, calcaneofibular ligament, and the posterior talofibular ligament, and although it is not directly associated with the ankle mortise, it too has been implicated in causes of ankle pathology that can lead to arthritic changes over time (**Fig. 2**).

Originally, it was thought that the ankle joint functioned much like a hinge, moving in one plane about a stationary transverse axis. However, Bottlang and colleagues[2] showed that the primary axis of the ankle is actually transmalleolar and is externally rotated about the lower leg ranging from 18° to 23°. Further studies built on this concept, demonstrating that the axis itself was not stationary, but in fact changed direction and orientation based on motion.[3] Coupled motion shown by the ability of the ankle to move in 3 planes about an axis that is constantly changing, occurs as the ankle is taken through its full range of motion. With dorsiflexion, the ankle joint axis rotates externally and everts, whereas the opposite internal and inversion motion occurs with plantarflexion. Furthermore, these coupled motions are controlled and stabilized by the medial and lateral collateral ligament complex and normal joint mobility occurs by gliding of articular surfaces and the rotation of the ligaments about their individual axes.[3]

The shape of the talus also plays a role in affecting coupled motion. The talus looks much like that of a wedge when visualized from above. The narrower posterior aspect of the talus sits within the mortise and couples sagittal and transverse plan motion providing approximately 4° of internal rotation while in a plantarflexed position. When in a dorsiflexed position, the wider anterior aspect of the talus is accommodated by the ankle syndesmosis and is able to externally rotate an average of 7°.[4] The ability of the newer, less constrained, more versatile generation of TAR devices to accommodate coupled motion in the ankle may be partly responsible for an increase in better surgical outcomes in the literature.

INDICATIONS AND PATIENT SELECTION

Although debate regarding indications and contraindications for TAR remain present within the literature, there appears to be a shift in thinking among foot and ankle surgeons loosening their restrictions of acceptable patient populations for ankle arthroplasty. Strict patient selection criteria has always been an expectation to predict good outcomes. Age, weight, smoking status, diabetes mellitus (DM), activity level,

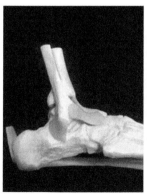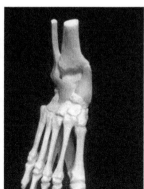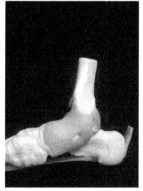

Fig. 2. Anteroposterior, lateral, and medial views of ankle ligament complex, showing the structures responsible for ankle stability.

and degree of adjacent joint arthritis have all been considered important criteria when choosing a good surgical candidate. Historically, the ideal surgical candidate for TAR was a middle-aged (>50 years old), nonobese, less active, non-DM, nonsmoker patient with no adjacent joint arthritis and minimal rear-foot deformity.[5] However, recent research has begun to increase the indications and expand the guidelines for patient populations that could be successful TAR candidates.

A primary concern when discussing the age of a TAR candidate is longevity of implant survivorship. Primary degenerative joint disease tends to affect older patients later in life, as it is less common in the ankle than the hip or knee.[6] However, because posttraumatic arthritis is more common in the ankle than other joints, it has a tendency to affect younger patient populations, giving rise to the need for definitive surgical intervention at an earlier decade of life.[7] The concern for the need for revision surgery due to implant failure in young patients stems from the idea that younger patients are more active and more likely to increase wear on the implant, leading to failure earlier than older individuals. Spirt and colleagues[8] supported this notion in their research, finding that patients younger than 54 years who underwent TAR, were 1.45 times more likely to need revision surgery and had a 2.65 times greater chance of implant failure than older patients. This information suggests that ankle arthrodesis may provide better long-term results for the younger patient population.

However, quality of life also must be a factor in the decision-making process as it relates to age and time of TAR treatment. Saltzman and colleagues[9] demonstrated that patients with end-stage ankle arthritis generally perceived a quality of life consistent with that of patients with end-stage renal failure and congestive heart disease, independent of age. Furthermore, newer research by Rodrigues-Pinto and colleagues[10] looking at the less constrained, modern fixed-bearing prosthesis compared TAR in older and younger patient populations, finding that patients younger than 50 demonstrated a better postoperative American Orthopaedic Foot and Ankle Society score and similar rates of complication and implant survivorship as those older than 50. Further research by Demetracopoulos and colleagues[7] not only found similar rates of revision surgery between younger and older patient populations who underwent TAR, but also found that patients younger than 55 who required revision surgery were much more likely to tolerate revision with a new TAR implant versus those older than 55. A younger patient may require an implant to last longer and also may be at a higher risk for wear failure; however, patient age alone may not directly correlate with activity level, suggesting the possibility of improving quality of life in a younger patient population using TARs.

Weight, and more specifically obesity, also has been a factor in patient selection for TAR surgery. Obesity is a multifactorial disease consisting of behavioral decisions, environmental factors, and genetic predisposition, and has been associated with increased risk of many chronic medical disorders.[11] The increased risk of medical comorbidities associated with obese patient populations, often presents a challenge surgically. Although long-term outcomes and complication rates for obese patients who undergo TAR remain unclear in the literature, the slightly higher revision and complication rates in total hip and knee surgery has been well documented,[12] suggesting that these patients would not be good candidates because of the detrimental effect of obesity on the musculoskeletal system. Obese patients may cause increased strain and wear on the implant components, leading to higher likelihood of earlier implant failure. However, Barg and colleagues[13] evaluated patients with TAR with a body mass index (BMI) greater than 30 and longer than 5 years of follow-up, demonstrating that all patients had a significant improvement in range of motion

(ROM) and pain and function scores, and similar implant survivorship of nonobese patients. Furthermore, a study by Gross and colleagues[14] looked at the effect of obesity by using different BMI scores on functional outcomes and complications with third-generation TAR and found similar results, indicating that obesity alone was not a significant risk factor for increased likelihood of revision or complications in TAR surgery.

The deleterious effects of active tobacco use, as it relates to increased postoperative complications and poor wound healing, has been well documented within the literature. This transcends multiple orthopedic fields and has been supported in arthroplasty, fracture healing, and wound-healing research.[15–17] Most recently Lampley and colleagues[18] evaluated complications and outcomes in TAR for smokers, nonsmokers, and former smokers and found that active smokers during the perioperative period had a significantly higher rate of wound complications and need for revision when compared with nonsmokers independent of other comorbidities. They further found that there was no significant difference in revision requirements or wound healing comparing former smokers with nonsmokers, indicating the significance of cessation of smoking before TAR surgery. Furthermore, other studies have shown active smoker populations to have lower implant survivorship in hip and knee replacement,[15,16] suggesting that this would likely be the same in TAR.

DM continues to be a serious growing health concern throughout the world, particularly among surgical candidates, as it has been shown to be associated with poor wound healing and perioperative complications.[19] Historically, DM with neuropathy has been a strong contraindication in TAR surgery.[20] Much of the research on complications with DM and arthroplasty surgery is extrapolated from hip and knee research. DM association with increased complication rates in ankle fractures is also well documented in the literature.[21] However, recent research by Gross and colleagues[22] regarding outcomes of TAR in patients with DM found no statistically significant difference in complication, revision, or failure rates and similar functional scores as the non-DM cohort. Gross and colleagues[22] also found that although differences in functional scores, complication rates, and revision surgery did not reach statistical significance, the patients with diabetes did have more complex revision surgeries. Much of current research is in its infancy and associated with short-term follow-up. However, it may suggest that TAR, as a treatment for end-stage arthritis in patients with well-controlled DM, could be effective in providing pain relief and better functional outcomes with similar rates of complications and revisions as their non-DM counterparts.

One other factor regarding patient selection and indications that has historically been a relative contraindication for TAR is degenerative changes in adjacent joints. The rationale was that TAR could create abnormal strain on the ankle and lead to further breakdown of the ankle implant. However, current research suggests that patients with combined rear-foot and ankle joint arthritis may benefit from TAR as compared with ankle arthrodesis. TAR decreases abnormal loads on the ankle. This leads to a decrease in loading to adjacent joints, thus decreasing degenerative changes, which is the opposite of ankle arthrodesis.[5] This thought process suggests TAR can be beneficial in patient populations with a combination of ankle and early-stage subtalar joint arthritis, provided that TAR increases ROM at the ankle joint and thus decreases stress across the subtalar joint. Using this treatment paradigm provides the ability to perform an isolated subtalar fusion concomitantly or at a later time based on clinical symptoms, the comfort level of the surgeon, and surgical needs of the patient (**Fig. 3**).

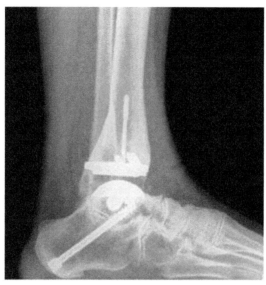

Fig. 3. Lateral view post-TAR in combination with primary fusion of subtalar joint.

PATIENT EVALUATION PREOPERATIVE PLANNING

The TAR patient population is becoming more diverse as outcomes continue to show improvement, and technology continues to create less constrained, more versatile implants. There are a few absolute contraindications, which include active infection, peripheral vascular disease, inadequate soft tissue coverage, and Charcot neuroarthropathy. Most patients in the TAR patient population present with a long history of continued degeneration of the ankle joint, either from posttraumatic pathology or affects from long-term abnormal joint biomechanics. Pain is often described as chronic and achy, and is increased with activity and weight-bearing and often decreased with rest. Most patients have already attempted much of the conservative treatment options available and failed alleviation of pain. Furthermore, many have already accepted a decreased activity load and are unable to carry out many of the activities they were once able to complete. It should be noted that not all patients who are referred to the senior authors (C.L.R. and A.M.S.) for TAR actually receive an ankle replacement. Identifying a good surgical candidate followed by an exhaustive preoperative evaluation is key to predicting good surgical outcomes.

Clinical evaluation is followed by imaging studies. The senior authors routinely order bilateral weight-bearing anteroposterior, lateral, and mortise views of the foot and ankle. Ancillary imaging studies that are also recommended are long leg calcaneal axial views, which allow evaluation of the subtalar joint and the rear-foot alignment (Cobey/Saltzman) view to determine any calcaneal, talus, or tibia pathology in the coronal plane. These views can help recognize the level of deformity (CORA) if any exists.[23] The long leg calcaneal axial view is created by using a larger 14 × 17-inch film sheet with the collimator focused at the subtalar joint in a 45° angle cephalad. The rear-foot alignment radiograph uses an elevated platform in combination with a 14 × 17-inch film placed 15° from vertical. The collimator is directed from a posterior to anterior direction perpendicular to the film and focused on the ankle joint. Ensuring realignment principles for foot and ankle surgery whereby the rear foot is aligned with the leg and the forefoot is aligned on the rear foot require particular angular relationships be measured in multiple anatomic planes. This allows for identification of any deformity or CORA. Computed tomography imaging is also used in surgical decision making.

In the frontal plane, the lateral distal tibial angle (LDTA), approximately 89° ± 3°, is measured using the ankle joint orientation line and the anatomic axis of the tibia. An abnormal increased or decreased LDTA is indicative of a valgus or varus distal tibia deformity, respectively. A valgus deformity is able to be compensated for by up to 30° of subtalar joint inversion, whereas a varus deformity is compensated by 15° of subtalar joint eversion. However, if the deformity is greater than subtalar joint compensation, or if the deformity forces maximum subtalar compensation in either direction, continued pathology in adjacent joints may become more symptomatic and should be corrected before TAR placement.

In the sagittal plane, the anterior distal tibial angle (ADTA) with a normal value of 80° ± 3° is formed by the mechanical axis of the tibia and the joint orientation line of the ankle. An increased or decreased value indicates a recurvatum or procurvatum deformity, respectively. Because the ankle usually has more plantarflexory ROM at approximately 50° than dorsiflexory ROM at approximately 20°, the ankle is able to likely completely compensate a recurvatum deforming force, rather than a procurvatum force. This also explains why a smaller procurvatum deforming force in the lower leg is often more symptomatic and more likely to require correction than a larger recurvatum deformity.

This is similar with frontal plane (varus/valgus) pathology, such that a larger decreased LDTA (valgus) is more likely to be completely compensated than a smaller increased LDTA (varus).[24] This is primarily why the senior authors feel that a valgus deformity that is not completely compensated is particularly challenging to correct before TAR placement. When malalignment is present and is not compensated for by adjacent joints, a potentially staged technique, including correction of deforming forces must be completed before TAR. This includes evaluation of adjacent soft tissue structures that can come under a great deal of tensioning forces with acute deformity correction. Allowing time for soft tissues to relax before TAR placement may need to be considered. As a general rule, malalignments and deforming forces in which the CORA is proximal (metaphyseal/diaphyseal) to the ankle joint, proximal osteotomies are indicated before TAR placement. Furthermore, in incongruent ankle joints (tibiotalar angle ≥10°), soft tissue balancing procedures must be combined with malalignment procedures. Finally, minimal distal tibia deformities (uncompensated ADTA/LDTA ≤10°) allow for realignment of deforming forces using a TAR device that provides the ability to alter the tibia slope of the cut **(Fig. 4)**.[25]

SURGICAL TECHNIQUE

The patient is placed on the operating table in the supine position. A blanket or bump is placed under the hip, centering the foot and ankle in a perpendicular position to the floor and a thigh tourniquet is applied to the ipsilateral extremity. The incision is made centered over the anterior ankle joint measuring approximately 10 to 12 cm in length. Identifying anatomic landmarks is imperative. The incision begins approximately 1 finger-width lateral to the tibial, is carried through the center point over the ankle joint between the transmalleolar axis and lateral to the tibialis anterior tendon and continues just beyond the talonavicular joint toward the second ray.

The incision is carried to the subcutaneous level, where all bleeders are bovied and cauterized as necessary. The superficial peroneal nerve is identified and protected

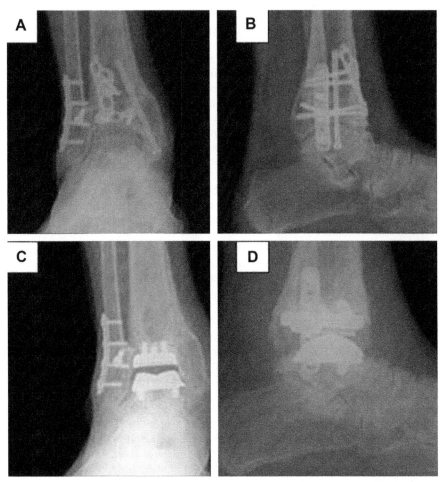

Fig. 4. Staged reconstruction. Anteroposterior and lateral views of supramalleolar osteotomy for correction of varus deformity before placement of TAR (*A, B*). Anteroposterior and lateral view of TAR placement months after supramalleolar osteotomy with noted correction of varus deformity and aligned ankle joint (*C, D*).

laterally. Once the anterior muscle tendons are identified, the anterior retinaculum is isolated, the neurovascular bundle is mobilized laterally and protected beneath the long extensor muscles and tendons. The capsule is incised, attempting to keep the tibialis anterior tendon within its tendon sheath. Separation and protection of the tibialis anterior tendon medially and retraction of the extensor hallucis and extensor digitorum longus tendons, along with the anterior tibial neurovascular bundle laterally, allows a full-thickness layer to be created as the surgeon approaches the ankle joint and distal tibial periosteum. The periosteal layer is then incised and elevated, allowing exposure to the ankle joint. The senior authors place great emphasis on the need for correct soft tissue balancing and ankle joint alignment during dissection, which will provide better anatomic placement of the tibial and talar components of the TAR. Careful debridement of any osteophytes, excessive synovial tissue or capsule, and clearance of the medial and lateral ankle gutters is completed.

Once dissection is complete, the tibial cut is completed accordingly, based on requirements needed to neutralize the ADTA and LDTA. Varus or valgus deformity ≤10° dictates whether to take more bone medially or laterally. Release of the deltoid ligament is sometimes needed to correct further talar tilt. The talar cut is then completed dependent or independent of the tibial cut based on the type of instrumentation used. Trial components are then positioned according to the surgical technique guide of the particular TAR implant being used, and ROM is tested. The goal is to have definitive component positioning in anatomic alignment without instability (**Figs. 5** and **6**). If this is not the case, further soft tissue balancing, including posterior tendon lengthening or ligamentous stability procedures may be needed based on cause of continued deformity. If hind-foot malalignment is present, rear-foot procedures discussed previously can be completed in combination with, or a staged technique before, TAR.

When only TAR and soft tissue procedures are completed with no boney fusions or osteotomies, the postoperative course entails immobilization in a posterior splint or cast, followed by removable walking boot for 4 to 6 weeks. Protected weight-bearing with crutches or walker after 2 weeks is generally allowed baring any complications. These guidelines are general and all dependent on incisional healing.

RESULTS/COMPLICATIONS AND A DISCUSSION MOVING FORWARD

It has been well documented that the most common denominator in the etiology of osteoarthritis in the ankle is posttraumatic causes.[26] Studies by Goldberg and colleagues[27] also have shown that the incidence of ankle fractures and ankle sprains often leading to posttraumatic ankle pain, continues to rise, suggesting that the demand for treatment of end-stage osteoarthritis by this patient population is also increasing. Although ankle arthrodesis has been the gold standard treatment for this patient population due to its success rates and reproducible outcomes, foot and ankle surgeons continue to expand the indications and use of TAR, showing that the newer, less constrained and more versatile implants provide similar results. A meta-analysis of the literature completed by Haddad and colleagues,[28] comparing intermediate outcomes of TAR and ankle fusion, demonstrated similar clinical scores, patient satisfaction, and revision rates for both treatment options. Further studies have echoed these results and shown a trend of increased utilization and decreased complication rates with TAR treatment for end-stage ankle arthritis.[29–31]

Complications are often divided into intraoperative versus postoperative and the postoperative category is often further broken down into major and minor findings. Intraoperative complications can range from medial or lateral malleolar fractures,

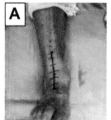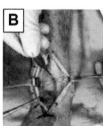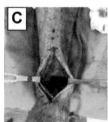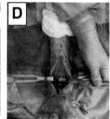

Fig. 5. Stages of surgical technique for TAR: anterior approach (*A*); retraction of neurovascular bundle laterally and maintaining protection of the tibialis anterior tendon within its tendon sheath (*B*); tibial and talar bone cuts complete (*C*); TAR implementation (*D*).

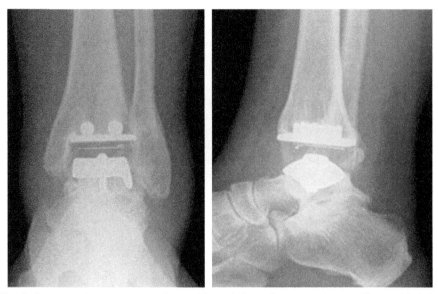

Fig. 6. Postoperative anteroposterior and lateral views demonstrating excellent ankle joint alignment after placement of TAR.

nonanatomic placement of the prosthetic implant, and undercorrection of soft tissue balancing often leading to instability. Although these complications are generally rare, the incidence of intraoperative complications decreases as the surgeon's learning curve increases.[30] In fact, Simonson and Roukis,[32] in a systemic review of the world literature on primary TAR, found an overall incidence of all types of complications, regardless of prosthesis system, was 44.2% during the surgeon's early learning curve period. Postoperative complications often include minor problems,

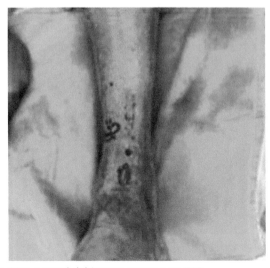

Fig. 7. Anterior incision wound dehiscence status post-TAR.

such as superficial infection and sensory neurapraxia, and more severe problems, such as deep infection, thromboembolic events, and need for revision surgery. Anecdotally, the most common postoperative complication in our experience, has been stiffness and/or tendonitis around the implant site. These are minor and often easily treated with physical therapy after the non–weight-bearing stage and a short course of anti-inflammatory medications. Incisional healing is by far the most worrisome step during the early postoperative period (**Fig. 7**). Furthermore, incisional complications not only effect TAR viability, but also postoperative protocols, thus potentially hindering long-term implant functionality.

SUMMARY

The goal of any TAR surgery is to improve function and decrease pain. It is important to spend a great deal of time preoperatively with the patient discussing every aspect of the surgical treatment plan and make a point to discuss patient expectations regarding end results. Furthermore, we follow evidence-based practices explaining to the patients that ROM in the ankle joint is expected to increase only 10° to 20°, as supported in the literature,[33] compared with preoperative values, and this plays a role in the decision-making process of TAR versus fusion. Survivorship of TAR remains controversial. Much of the data are level 3 or 4 studies often completed by inventors of different TAR systems. A recent meta-analysis by Zaidi and colleagues[33] found a 10-year survivorship of 89%, independent of the many different TAR systems, indicating great improvement in reliability with the newer generation implants. Complications are spelled out in our preoperative discussions. These include a discussion of both minor and major complications, such as explantation, excessive revisional surgery, and even amputation. TAR should no longer be considered a "fringe" or inferior procedure to ankle fusion, but rather a viable alternative in the right patient population. Steadfast rules and previous contraindications to TAR treatment are constantly being reevaluated, as new data continue to support expansion of TAR indications and an increase in surgical candidates from a more diverse patient population. Not all patients with end-stage ankle arthritis are candidates for a TAR procedure. Using an exhaustive knowledge of anatomy, biomechanics, and ankle joint pathology, in combination with careful patient selection and perioperative surgical planning based on the most current evidence available, is paramount to successful TAR outcome.

REFERENCES

1. Daniels TR, Alastair SE, Penner M, et al. Intermediate-term results of total ankle replacement and ankle arthrodesis. J Bone Joint Surg Am 2014;96(2):135–42.
2. Bottlang M, Marsh JL, Brown TD. Articulated external fixation of the ankle: minimizing motion resistance by accurate axis alignment. J Biomech 1999;32:63–70.
3. Leardini A, O'connor JJ, Catani F. A geometric model of the human ankle joint. J Biomech 1999;32:585–91.
4. Michelson JD, Helgemo SL Jr. Kinematics of the axially loaded ankle. Foot Ankle Int 1995;16(9):577–82.
5. Easley ME, Vertullo CJ, Urban WC, et al. Total ankle arthroplasty. J Am Acad Orthop Surg 2002;10(3):157–67.
6. Huch K, Kuettner KE, Dieppe P. Osteoarthritis in ankle and knee joints. Semin Arthritis Rheum 1997;26(4):667–74.
7. Demetracopoulos CA, Adams SB Jr, Queen RM, et al. Effect of age on outcomes in total ankle arthroplasty. Foot Ankle Int 2015;36(8):871–80.

8. Spirt AA, Assal M, Sigvard T, et al. Complications and failure after total ankle arthroplasty. J Bone Joint Surg 2004;86(6):1172–8.

9. Saltzman CL, Zimmerman MB, O'Rourke M, et al. Impact of comorbidities on the measurement of health in patients with ankle osteoarthritis. J Bone Joint Surg Am 2006;88(11):2366–72.

10. Rodrigues-Pinto R, Muras J, Martín Oliva X, et al. Total ankle replacement in patients under the age of 50: should the indications be revised? Foot Ankle Surg 2013;19(4):229–33.

11. Tjepkema M. Adult obesity. Health Rep 2006;17:9–25.

12. Guenther D, Schmidl S, Klatte TO, et al. Overweight and obesity in hip and knee arthroplasty: evaluation of 6078 cases. World J Orthop 2015;6:137–44.

13. Barg A, Knupp M, Anderson AE, et al. Total ankle replacement in obese patients: component stability, weight change, and functional outcome in 118 consecutive patients. Foot Ankle Int 2011;32(10):925–32.

14. Gross CE, Lampley A, Green CL, et al. The effect of obesity on functional outcomes and complications in total ankle arthroplasty. Foot Ankle Int 2016;37(2): 137–41.

15. Kapadia BH, Issa K, Pivec R, et al. Tobacco use may be associated with increased revision and complication rates following total hip arthroplasty. J Arthroplasty 2014;29(4):777–80.

16. Kapadia BH, Johnson AJ, Naziri Q, et al. Increased revision rates after total knee arthroplasty in patients who smoke. J Arthroplasty 2012;27(9):1690–5.

17. Mosely LH, Finseth F. Cigarette smoking: impairment of digital blood flow and wound healing in the hand. Hand 1977;9(2):97–101.

18. Lampley A, Gross CE, Green CL, et al. Association of cigarette use and complication rates and outcomes following total ankle arthroplasty. Foot Ankle Int 2016; 37(10):1052–9.

19. Tsang ST, Gaston P. Adverse peri-operative outcomes following elective total hip replacement in diabetes mellitus: a systematic review and meta-analysis of cohort studies. Bone Joint J 2013;95B(11):1474–9.

20. Chou LB, Coughlin MT, Hansen S Jr, et al. Osteoarthritis of the ankle: the role of arthroplasty. J Am Acad Orthop Surg 2008;16(5):249–59.

21. SooHoo NF, Krenek L, Eagan MJ, et al. Complication rates following open reduction and internal fixation of ankle fractures. J Bone Joint Surg Am 2009;91(5): 1042–9.

22. Gross CE, Green CL, DeOrio JK, et al. Impact of diabetes on outcomes of total ankle replacement. Foot Ankle Int 2015;36(10):1144–9.

23. Paley D. The correction of complex foot deformities using Ilizarov's distraction osteotomies. Clin Orthop 1993;293:97.

24. Mendicino RW, Catanzariti AR, Reeves CL. Percutaneous supramalleolar osteotomy for distal tibial (near articular) ankle deformities. J Am Podiatr Med Assoc 2005;95(1):72–84.

25. Bonasia DE, Dettoni F, Femino JE, et al. Total ankle replacement: why, when and how? Iowa Orthop J 2010;30:119–30.

26. Saltzman CL, Salamon ML, Blanchard GM, et al. Epidemiology of ankle arthritis: report of a consecutive series of 639 patients from a tertiary orthopaedic center. Iowa Orthop J 2005;25:44–6.

27. Goldberg AJ, Macgregor A, Dawson J, et al. The demand incidence of symptomatic ankle osteoarthritis presenting to foot & ankle surgeons in the United Kingdom. Foot Edinb 2012;22:163–6.

28. Haddad SL, Coetzee JC, Estok R, et al. Intermediate and long-term outcomes of total ankle arthroplasty and ankle arthrodesis. A systematic review of the literature. J Bone Joint Surg Am 2007;89(9):1899–905.

29. Stavrakis AI, SooHoo NF. Trends in complication rates following ankle arthrodesis and total ankle replacement. J Bone Joint Surg Am 2016;98(17):1453–8.

30. Raikin SM, Rasouli MR, Espandar R, et al. Trends in treatment of advanced ankle arthropathy by total ankle replacement or ankle fusion. Foot Ankle Int 2014;35(3):216–24.

31. Gougoulias N, Khanna A, Maffulli N. How successful are current ankle replacements? A systemic review of the literature [review]. Clin Orthop Relat Res 2010;468(1):199–208.

32. Simonson DC, Roukis TS. Incidence of complications during the surgeon learning curve period for primary total ankle replacement: a systematic review [review]. Clin Podiatr Med Surg 2015;32(4):473–82.

33. Zaidi R, Cro S, Gurusamy K, et al. The outcome of total ankle replacement: a systematic review and meta-analysis [review]. Bone Joint J 2013;95B(11):1500–7.

Complex Total Ankle Arthroplasty

Stephen A. Brigido, DPM[a],*, Scott C. Carrington, DPM[a],
Nicole M. Protzman, MS[b]

KEYWORDS

- Avascular necrosis • Malalignment of the ankle • Total ankle replacement
- Valgus ankle deformity • Varus ankle deformity

KEY POINTS

- With continued evolution in implant design and improved techniques, the indications for total ankle replacement continue to expand.
- Thorough preoperative planning and a meticulous surgical technique are paramount to achieving good outcomes in complex total ankle replacement cases.
- Research has confirmed that preoperative deformities can be addressed at the time of prosthesis implantation with results comparable to neutrally aligned ankles.
- Avascular necrosis no longer represents an absolute contraindication to total ankle replacement.

INTRODUCTION

Despite the high failure rates associated with first-generation ankle implants,[1–5] continued evolution in implant design and refined surgical techniques have produced marked improvements in outcomes.[6–8] Studies comparing arthrodesis and total ankle replacement (TAR) have demonstrated similar improvements in pain and functionality,[6–8] and others have shown that TAR offers the added benefits of maintaining range of motion, restoring normal kinematics, and limiting adjacent joint degeneration.[9–11]

With superior implants and an increased understanding of ligamentous balancing and component alignment, the indications for TAR continue to expand to include cases of increasing complexity.[12,13] In fact, many factors once considered relative

Disclosure Statement: Dr S.A. Brigido serves on the surgery advisory board for Alliqua. He also serves as a consultant for Stryker. Alliqua and Stryker had no knowledge or influence in study design, protocol, or data collection.

[a] Foot and Ankle Reconstruction, Foot and Ankle Department, Coordinated Health, 2775 Schoenersville Road, Bethlehem, PA 18017, USA; [b] Clinical Integration Department, Coordinated Health, 3435 Winchester Road, Allentown, PA 18104, USA
* Corresponding author.
E-mail address: drsbrigido@mac.com

or absolute contraindications can now be successfully addressed at the time of prosthesis implantation or in a staged fashion.

Even though malalignment is commonly encountered with end-stage ankle arthritis, significant preoperative varus and valgus deformities (>10°) have historically been considered a relative contraindication.[14,15] In the presence of a preexisting deformity, uneven stress distributions can give way to aseptic loosening, edge loading, and premature implant failure.[14,15] More recent studies, however, have shown that a stable, plantigrade foot can be obtained with appropriate ligament balancing, correction of associated deformities, and replacement of the ankle joint.[16–18]

Avascular necrosis (AVN) of the talus has also been considered an absolute contraindication for TAR,[19–22] given the potential for talar component subsidence and early implant failure.[19,20] However, AVN has become much less of a concern with newer prosthetic designs that provide increased surface coverage of the talus,[13] and with the recent introduction of custom-made long-stem components capable of incorporating into the calcaneus and replacing the body of the talus,[23] complete AVN is no longer considered a contraindication by many surgeons.[13]

Within, complex TAR cases are discussed, detailing the preoperative planning process as well as the techniques needed to achieve a stable TAR.

PATIENT EVALUATION OVERVIEW

A firm understanding of the patient's deformity is necessary to achieve the best possible outcome. The physical examination should include a thorough weight-bearing and non-weight-bearing examination. During the weight-bearing examination, the surgeon should assess the position of the ankle relative to the extremity and take note of the position of the heel, mid foot, and forefoot. The surgeon should assess proximal leg and knee deformity as well, including genu varum and valgus and any femoral or hip disorders. Evaluating the position of the proximal leg, knee, and thigh will allow the surgeon to understand the mechanical axis of the extremity, which will assist with intraoperative positioning of the implant. During the non-weight-bearing examination, the surgeon should take note of any peritalar arthritis as well as the mobility of the subtalar and midtarsal joints. The mobility of the peritalar joints will dictate whether additional bony procedures will need to be performed. It is the surgeon's preference as to when these additional procedures are performed. The authors prefer to stage procedures, such as subtalar and talonavicular arthrodeses. This method allows total ankle patients to enter physical therapy as soon as the sutures are removed from the skin. They will, however, often perform osseous procedures, such as calcaneal slide osteotomies, at the time of TAR.

Weight-bearing ankle radiographs should be a routine part of the preoperative evaluation. In the setting of deformity, the weight-bearing radiographs allow the surgeon to assess whether the varus or valgus deformity is congruent or incongruent. Incongruent varus and valgus deformities are defined as those with talar tilt on a weight-bearing radiograph of more than 10° in either direction.[24] Advanced imaging, such as MRI and computed tomography, are also routinely used as part of the preoperative evaluation. These imaging modalities allow the surgeon to assess subchondral bone cysts and periarticular soft tissue structures, such as the deltoid ligament, lateral collateral ligaments, and tendons. Understanding the viability of these structures is important for intraoperative balancing in the setting of deformity.

THE VARUS ARTHRITIC ANKLE

Of the frontal plane deformities, the varus ankle is widely considered the more manageable deformity to treat. As mentioned in the previous section, the surgeon must consider whether the deformity is congruent (<10° tibiotalar malalignment) (**Fig. 1**) or incongruent (>10° tibiotalar malalignment) (**Fig. 2**). Congruent varus ankles are usually due to the talus driving into the tibia. They may have some lateral ligamentous instability and some medial deltoid tightness. When treating the congruent varus ankle, a deltoid peel is performed. By removing the deep deltoid from the talus with a surgical blade or elevator, talar alignment is restored relative to the tibia. Care must be taken to get to the posterior deltoid and the posterior tibial tendon sheath. The sheath of the posterior tibial tendon often needs to be released, because this may be a point of adhesion preventing the talus from being reduced into alignment. Sizing with the appropriate polyethylene component will ensure tensioning/balancing of the lateral collateral ligament structures. It is rare in the authors' experience to have to reconstruct the lateral ligaments in a congruent varus ankle.

The incongruent varus ankle may require more work to restore the tibiotalar alignment. A deep deltoid peel is still incorporated, but often needs to be augmented with a vertical malleolar osteotomy, as described by Doets and colleagues.[25] This osteotomy allows the medial malleolus to slide distally, taking the tension off of the medial side of the ankle. This technique is performed when the polyethylene component is being sized, to ensure proper balancing of the ankle joint. When this osteotomy is performed, it is often necessary to lengthen the posterior tibial tendon, release the sheath of the posterior tendon, and tighten the lateral ligament structures. Again, each

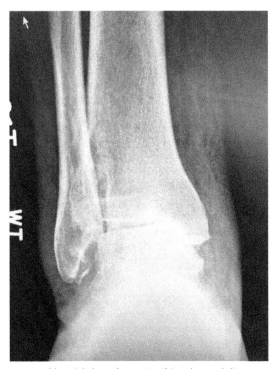

Fig. 1. Congruent varus ankle with less than 10° tibiotalar malalignment.

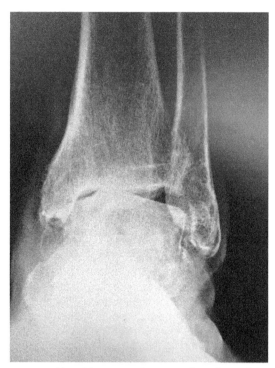

Fig. 2. Incongruent varus ankle with greater than 10° tibiotalar malalignment.

of these procedures is performed while the polyethylene component is being sized to ensure proper balancing.

When soft tissue balancing has been performed and the bone structures remain mechanically malaligned, it may be necessary to incorporate osteotomies or fusions during the TAR or in a staged fashion. In the setting of distal tibial malposition, the principles of limb deformity and CORA (center of rotation and angulation) must be followed. In severe cases of distal tibial deformity, the supramalleolar osteotomy can be performed to restore the mechanical alignment to the limb. In cases where the tibial alignment is maintained, but foot alignment is poor, procedures, such as hindfoot fusions and osteotomies (eg, calcaneal slide), may be used to restore the position of the foot relative to the leg and ground and to eliminate edge loading stress across the prosthetic.

Although rarely encountered in the authors' experience, tendon transfers may be used to help augment the repair of an incongruent varus ankle. The 2 most common tendon transfers used are the posterior tibial tendon to peroneus brevis tendon and the flexor hallucis longs to the fifth metatarsal. These tendon transfers can support the correction of the deformity in a dynamic fashion, but can be technically challenging to perform.

THE VALGUS ARTHRITIC ANKLE

Correcting the arthritic valgus ankle can be one of the more challenging procedures that a foot and ankle surgeon can perform. Similar to the varus joint, the surgeon must first recognize whether the joint is congruent valgus (**Fig. 3**) or incongruent valgus (**Fig. 4**). It is the authors' experience that the valgus ankle is more commonly

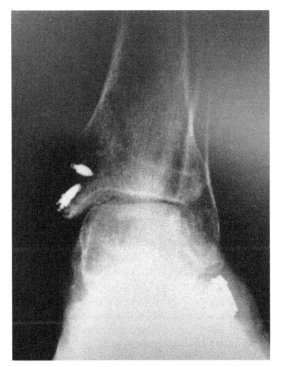

Fig. 3. Congruent valgus ankle with less than 10° tibiotalar malalignment.

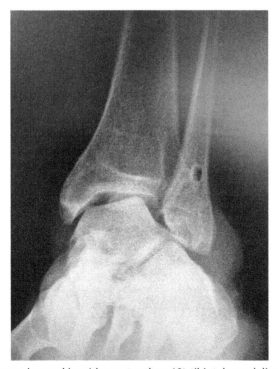

Fig. 4. Incongruent valgus ankle with greater than 10° tibiotalar malalignment.

incongruent, and with that comes an insufficient deltoid ligament, and in many instances, a short fibula. Although the release of the deltoid ligament is the cornerstone to the successful treatment of the varus ankle, the valgus ankle produces an incompetent deltoid ligament that needs to be tensioned appropriately with polyethylene sizing. If the deltoid ligament needs to be reconstructed, the authors prefer to perform the deltoid ligament advancement in a staged procedure before the TAR. While performing the TAR, the lateral soft tissue structures often need to be released from the lateral talus and distal fibula.

The surgeon also must assess the length of the fibula as well as the position of the hind foot and mid foot in relation to the ground and leg. In the setting of significant valgus, a short fibula must often be lengthened with a Z-lengthening osteotomy (**Fig. 5**). In many instances, the surgeon may find that staged subtalar and talonavicular fusions will help create a plantargrade foot before treating the arthritic valgus ankle.

The authors have found that it is far more difficult to achieve long-term survivorship in the valgus ankle compared with the neutral or varus ankle. The role of the incompetent deltoid ligament presents a unique challenge to the foot and ankle surgeon. The deltoid ligament is extremely difficult and unpredictable to reconstruct, and far too often, surgeons new to ankle arthroplasty will try to "balance" the joint by using an oversized polyethylene component. When the polyethylene component is oversized, the joint line of the ankle is moved distally, which changes the biomechanics of the joint and may cause excessive polyethylene wear with resultant aseptic loosening of the prosthetic, and ultimately, subsidence of one or more of the prosthetic components.

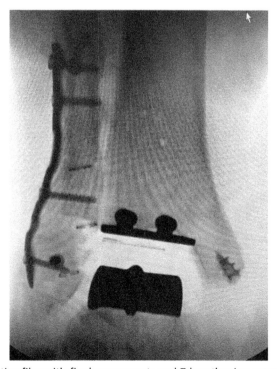

Fig. 5. Postoperative film with final components and Z-lengthening osteotomy.

ANKLE ARTHROPLASTY WITH TALAR AVASCULAR NECROSIS

Total ankle arthroplasty in the setting of AVN of the talus presents a unique challenge to the foot and ankle surgeon. A stable bone-implant interface is critical for the successful outcome of ankle arthroplasty. Unlike the hip and knee, the ankle joint has far less bone stock available to accept a prosthetic component, so any compromise to the viability of underlying bone must be investigated. Recent advancements in component design and trial and error have demonstrated that arthroplasty with talar AVN can be successful.

When considering TAR in a patient with a history of talar AVN, the surgeon must assess the extent of AVN involvement and the percentage of viable bone, as this will guide clinical decision making (**Fig. 6**). If AVN is limited to the superior portion of the talar body and can be eliminated with the talar bone cut, ankle arthroplasty can be performed. If AVN extends below the level of the superior border of the talar neck, arthrodesis may be advisable.[26] The authors prefer arthrodesis in the latter scenario.

In the presence of nonviable bone, subsidence of the talar component is inevitable given the lack of structural support. However, successful TAR can be performed when the implant is sufficiently supported (**Fig. 7**).[27,28] Lee and colleagues[27] presented 2 cases where revascularized talar bodies underwent successful mobile bearing TAR. The results suggest that necrotic bone healing to the upper border of the talar neck provides adequate support for a talar component.[27] More recently, Devalia and colleagues[28] demonstrated the success of a 2-staged approach where subtalar joint arthrodesis was followed by TAR to address arthritis and AVN of the talus. The investigators concluded that subtalar joint arthrodesis improved talar vascularity and

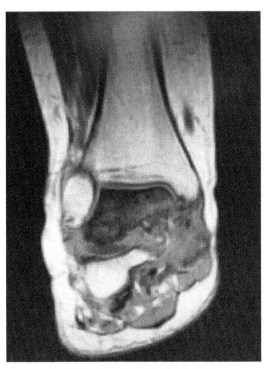

Fig. 6. T1-weighted image revealing extensive talar body AVN.

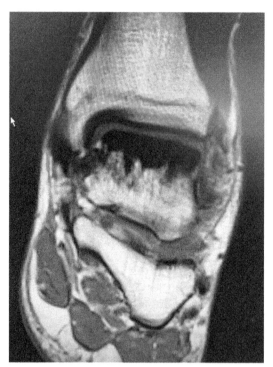

Fig. 7. T1-weighted image showing superior talar body necrosis.

increased the success of TAR in this cohort. Although limited to 3-year follow-up, the study presents a promising option when faced with osteonecrosis.

In a talus with compromised vascularity, there is a risk of damaging the remaining blood supply with TAR implantation.[29,30] Oppermann and colleagues[30] mapped out the microvascular supply of the talus and demonstrated the negative influence of chamfered components on the deep talar body blood supply. When performing TAR in patients with AVN, flat-cut talar components that are able to resect necrotic bone without violating the deep vasculature should be considered.

In cases of advanced talar AVN, viable options for primary and revisional TAR have been demonstrated. Schuberth and colleagues[31] had good results when reinforcing the talar body with metallic rods and bone cement augmentation. Short-term success has also been reported with the use of a total talar prosthesis for a failed TAR with talar collapse.[32]

Osteonecrosis of the talus presents many challenges to the success of TAR. However, when tibiotalar adjacent joint arthritis is present, all efforts should be made to preserve the ankle joint. Reasonable alternatives to arthrodesis have been reported in this setting. Careful planning and proper imaging of the ankle can lead to successful outcomes with joint replacement.

SUMMARY

The evolution of current generation total ankle prosthetics has afforded many patients suffering from end stage degenerative joint disease of the ankle the opportunity to function with decreased pain and improved function. Although prosthetic guidance, instrumentation, and education have all improved greatly over the last 30 years, both surgeons and patients can experience significant complications when ankle deformity is not managed correctly. The authors follow a rigid protocol to address frontal plane deformity and AVN.

In the setting of incongruent varus, TAR is performed irrespective of the size of the deformity, as long as the following criteria are met:

1. The foot is able to be reduced/corrected back to a neutral, plantigrade foot.
2. The bone quality of the joint is sufficient to support a prosthetic long term.
3. Any periarticular soft tissue structural damage can be repaired either at the time of ankle replacement or in a staged fashion.

The valgus ankle does not grant the same freedom as the neutral or varus ankle. If the valgus ankle has become incongruent, patients are typically limited to ankle arthrodesis. The exception includes patients who have a mild incongruent valgus that can be reconstructed into a congruent valgus or neutral ankle in a staged fashion.

As described in the previous section, AVN presents its own unique challenges. The introduction of a "flat top talar" component allows surgeons to perform TAR in select AVN cases. When AVN is limited to the superior portion of the talar body, the surgeon can remove compromised bone with the talar cut and proceed with prosthesis implantation. Given the results of Oppermann and colleagues,[30] the investigators do not advocate a chamfered talar component for patients with talar body AVN, but rather a flat-cut talar component that avoids violating the deep vasculature. Finally, patients who have talar body AVN that extends below the level of the superior border of the talar neck are excluded from ankle arthroplasty.

Foot and ankle surgeons who are performing arthroplasty should become confident and comfortable with patients suffering from neutral joint arthritis and progressively increase to patients suffering from frontal plane deformity. In line with this recommendation, the authors suggest starting with the varus ankle and progressing to cases of increasing complexity. Sound clinical judgment should be exercised when dealing with AVN of the talus.

REFERENCES

1. Helm R, Stevens J. Long-term results of total ankle replacement. J Arthroplasty 1986;1:271–7. Available at: https://www.ncbi.nlm.nih.gov/pubmed/3559603.
2. Kirkup J. Richard Smith ankle arthroplasty. J R Soc Med 1985;78:301–4. Available at: https://www.ncbi.nlm.nih.gov/pmc/articles/PMC1289679/pdf/jrsocmed00210-0030.pdf.
3. Herberts P, Goldie IF, Körner L, et al. Endoprosthetic arthroplasty of the ankle joint. A clinical and radiological follow-up. Acta Orthop Scand 1982;53:687–96. Available at: http://www.tandfonline.com/doi/pdf/10.3109/17453678208992277.
4. Lachiewicz PF. Total ankle arthroplasty. Indications, techniques, and results. Orthop Rev 1994;23:315–20. Available at: https://www.ncbi.nlm.nih.gov/pubmed/8008441.
5. Stauffer RN, Segal NM. Total ankle arthroplasty: four years' experience. Clin Orthop Relat Res 1981;160:217–21. Available at: http://journals.lww.com/corr/Citation/1981/10000/Total_Ankle_Arthroplasty__Four_Years__Experience_.32.aspx.
6. Haddad SL, Coetzee JC, Estok R, et al. Intermediate and long-term outcomes of total ankle arthroplasty and ankle arthrodesis. A systematic review of the

literature. J Bone Joint Surg Am 2007;89:1899–905. Available at: http://www. orthopedicsmagazine.com/foundation/documents/new/JBJS%20AM%202007 %20Haddad%20Coetzee-%20Intermed%20and%20Long%20term%20outcomes %20of%20TAA%20and%20Ankle%20Arthrodesis.pdf.

7. Kim HJ, Suh DH, Yang JH, et al. Total ankle arthroplasty versus ankle arthrodesis for the treatment of end-stage ankle arthritis: a meta-analysis of comparative studies. Int Orthop 2017;41(1):101–9. Available at: http://link.springer.com/ article/10.1007%2Fs00264-016-3303-3.

8. van Heiningen J, Vliet Vlieland TP, van der Heide HJ. The mid-term outcome of total ankle arthroplasty and ankle fusion in rheumatoid arthritis: a systematic review. BMC Musculoskelet Disord 2013;14:306. Available at: https://www.ncbi. nlm.nih.gov/pmc/articles/PMC4231459/pdf/1471-2474-14-306.pdf.

9. Pedowitz DI, Kane JM, Smith GM, et al. Total ankle arthroplasty versus ankle arthrodesis: a comparative analysis of arc of movement and functional outcomes. Bone Joint J 2016;98B:634–40. Available at: http://www.bjj.boneandjoint.org.uk/ content/98-B/5/634.long.

10. Singer S, Klejman S, Pinsker E, et al. Ankle arthroplasty and ankle arthrodesis: gait analysis compared with normal controls. J Bone Joint Surg Am 2013;95: e191(1-10). Available at: http://jbjs.org/content/95/24/e191.long.

11. SooHoo NF, Zingmond DS, Ko CY. Comparison of reoperation rates following ankle arthrodesis and total ankle arthroplasty. J Bone Joint Surg Am 2007;89: 2143–9. Available at: http://jbjs.org/content/89/10/2143.long.

12. Gougoulias N, Maffulli N. Osteotomies for managing varus and valgus malalignment with total ankle replacement. Clin Podiatr Med Surg 2015;32:529–42. Available at: https://www.clinicalkey.com/#!/content/playContent/1-s2.0-S0891842 215000555?returnurl=http:%2F%2Flinkinghub.elsevier.com%2Fretrieve%2Fpii% 2FS0891842215000555%3Fshowall%3Dtrue&referrer=.

13. Myerson M, Christensen JC, Steck JK, et al. Avascular necrosis of the foot and ankle. Foot Ankle Spec 2012;5:128–36. Available at: http://fas.sagepub.com/ content/5/2/128.extract.

14. Doets HC, Brand R, Nelissen RG. Total ankle arthroplasty in inflammatory joint disease with use of two mobile-bearing designs. J Bone Joint Surg Am 2006; 88:1272–84. Available at: http://jbjs.org/content/88/6/1272.long.

15. Woods PL, Deakin S. Total ankle replacement. The results in 200 ankles. J Bone Joint Surg Br 2003;85:334–41. Available at: http://www.bjj.boneandjoint.org.uk/ content/85-B/3/334.long.

16. Kim BS, Lee JW. Total ankle replacement for the varus unstable osteoarthritic ankle. Tech Foot Ankle Surg 2010;9:157–64. Available at: http://journals.lww.com/ techfootankle/Abstract/2010/12000/Total_Ankle_Replacement_for_the_Varus_ Unstable.3.aspx.

17. Knupp M, Stufkens SA, Bolliger LM, et al. Total ankle replacement and supramalleolar osteotomies for malaligned osteoarthritic ankles. Tech Foot Ankle Surg 2010;9:175–81. Available at: http://journals.lww.com/techfootankle/Abstract/ 2010/12000/Total_Ankle_Replacement_and_Supramalleolar.5.aspx.

18. Karantana A, Hobson S, Dhar S. The Scandinavian total ankle replacement: survivorship at 5 and 8 years comparable to other series. Clin Orthop Relat Res 2010;468:951–7. Available at: https://www.ncbi.nlm.nih.gov/pmc/articles/ PMC2835582/pdf/11999_2009_Article_971.pdf.

19. Stamatis ED, Myerson MS. How to avoid specific complications of total ankle replacement. Foot Ankle Clin 2002;7:765–89. Available at: https://www.ncbi. nlm.nih.gov/pubmed/12516733.

20. Raikin SM, Myerson MS. Avoiding and managing complications of the Agility total ankle replacement system. Orthopedics 2006;29:930–8. Available at: https://www.ncbi.nlm.nih.gov/pubmed/17061420.

21. Guyer AJ, Richardson G. Current concepts review: total ankle arthroplasty. Foot Ankle Int 2008;29:256–64. Available at: http://fai.sagepub.com/content/29/2/256.long.

22. Murnaghan JM, Warnock DS, Henderson SA. Total ankle replacement. Early experiences with STAR prosthesis. Ulster Med J 2005;74:9–13. Available at: https://www.ncbi.nlm.nih.gov/pmc/articles/PMC2475487/pdf/ulstermedj00001-0012.pdf.

23. Myerson MS, Won HY. Primary and revision total ankle replacement using custom-designed prostheses. Foot Ankle Clin 2008;13:521–38, x. Available at: http://www.sciencedirect.com/science/article/pii/S1083751508000508.

24. Trincat S, Kouyoumdjian P, Asencio G. Total ankle arthroplasty and coronal plane deformities. Orthop Traumatol Surg Res 2012;98:75–84. Available at: http://www.sciencedirect.com/science/article/pii/S1877051711008070.

25. Doets HC, van der Plaat LW, Klein JP. Medial malleolar osteotomy for the correction of varus deformity during total ankle arthroplasty: results in 15 ankles. Foot Ankle Int 2008;29:171–7. Available at: http://fai.sagepub.com/content/29/2/171.long.

26. Tenenbaum S, Stockton KG, Bariteau T, et al. Salvage of avascular necrosis of the talus by combined ankle and hindfoot arthrodesis without structural bone graft. Foot Ankle Int 2015;36:282–7. Available at: http://fai.sagepub.com/content/36/3/282.long.

27. Lee KB, Cho SG, Jung ST, et al. Total ankle arthroplasty following revascularization of avascular necrosis of the talar body: two case reports and literature review. Foot Ankle Int 2008;29:852–8. Available at: http://fai.sagepub.com/content/29/8/852.long.

28. Devalia KL, Ramaskandhan J, Muthumayandi K, et al. Early results of a novel technique: hindfoot fusion in talus osteonecrosis prior to ankle arthroplasty: a case series. Foot (Edinb) 2015;25:200–5.

29. Tennant JN, Rungprai C, Pizzimenti MA, et al. Risks to the blood supply of the talus with four methods of total ankle arthroplasty: a cadaveric injection study. J Bone Joint Surg Am 2014;96:395–402. Available at: http://www.jbjs.org/cgi/pmidlookup?view=long&pmid=24599201.

30. Oppermann J, Franzen J, Spies C, et al. The microvascular anatomy of the talus: a plastination study on the influence of total ankle replacement. Surg Radiol Anat 2014;36:487–94. Available at: http://link.springer.com/article/10.1007%2Fs00276-013-1219-9.

31. Schuberth JM, Christensen JC, Rialson JA. Metal-reinforced cement augmentation for complex talar subsidence in failed total ankle arthroplasty. J Foot Ankle Surg 2011;50:766–72. Available at: http://www.jfas.org/article/S1067-2516(11)00381-4/fulltext.

32. Tsukamoto S, Tanaka Y, Maegawa N, et al. Total talar replacement following collapse of the talar body as a complication of total ankle arthroplasty: a case report. J Bone Joint Surg Am 2010;92:2115–20. Available at: http://jbjs.org/content/92/11/2115.long.

Revision Total Ankle Arthroplasty

Jerome K. Steck, DPM[a],*, John M. Schuberth, DPM[b],
Jeffrey C. Christensen, DPM[c,d], Cynthia A. Luu, DPM[e]

KEYWORDS

- Ankle surgery • Total ankle arthroplasty • Revision TAA • TAA complications

KEY POINTS

- Total ankle arthroplasty (TAA) is a difficult procedure with a high learning curve.
- Revision TAA is even more demanding and requires experienced surgeons to undertake.
- The principles for revision are as follows: ensure infection is eradicated; ensure alignment; fill resultant defect with a combination of implant, bone graft, and possibly cement to provide stability to revisional implant; and to correct cause of failure.

INTRODUCTION

Over the past 2 decades, improvements in total ankle implant design, materials, and surgical technique have led to better functional outcomes. However, known complications inherent to total joint replacement remain that may require revisional surgery. Glazebrook and colleagues[1] found 9 main complications in the literature: intraoperative fracture, postoperative fracture, wound healing problems, deep infection, aseptic loosening, nonunion, implant failure, subsidence, and technical error. They proposed a classification system based on the rate of failure for a given complication. Intraoperative bone fracture and wound healing problems are considered low grade and very unlikely to cause failure. Technical error, subsidence, and postoperative bone fracture are classified as medium-grade and lead to failure less

Disclosure: Dr J.K. Steck is a consultant for Zimmer Biomet, Wright Medical, Stryker, and Integra. Dr J.M. Schuberth is on the STAR advisory board. Dr J.C. Christensen is a consultant for Stryker, Wright Medical, and Paragon 28. Dr C.A. Luu reports no commercial interests or potential conflicts of interest.
[a] Southern Arizona Orthopedics, 6567 East Carondolet Drive, Suite 415, Tucson, AZ 85710, USA; [b] Foot and Ankle Surgery, Department of Orthopedic Surgery, Kaiser San Francisco Medical Center, Kaiser Foundation Hospital, French Campus, 450, 6th Avenue, San Francisco, CA 94118, USA; [c] Podiatric Section, Department of Orthopedics, Swedish Medical Center, Seattle, WA, USA; [d] Ankle & Foot Clinics Northwest, 3131 Nassau Street, Suite 101, Everett, WA 98201, USA; [e] Tucson Medical Center, Midwestern University, 5301 East Grant Road, Tucson, AZ 85712, USA
* Corresponding author.
E-mail address: jsteck@acssurgeons.com

Clin Podiatr Med Surg 34 (2017) 541–564
http://dx.doi.org/10.1016/j.cpm.2017.05.010
0891-8422/17/© 2017 Elsevier Inc. All rights reserved.

podiatric.theclinics.com

than 50% of the time. Deep infection, aseptic loosening, and implant failure are considered high grade and lead to failure of total ankle arthroplasty (TAA) more than 50% of the time.

In total ankle surgery, it is generally accepted that revision constitutes manipulation of one or more of the metal components.[2–4] Henricson and colleagues[2] reviewed the literature to provide a consensus on the definition and defined revisional TAA as exchange or removal of one or more of the components except incidental exchange of the polyethylene meniscus. In their study on the Agility total ankle, Knecht and colleagues[3] differentiated major revisions from secondary procedures. They considered major revisions as any procedure requiring removal or replacement of one or both of the metal components. Secondary minor procedures included any procedure of the foot and ankle related to the total ankle replacement, such as calcaneal osteotomies, subtalar fusions, and ankle ligament augmentation. In the primary author's experience with 400 Agility total ankle arthroplasties with 1-year to 6-year follow-up, the major and minor complication rate was 8% and 14%, respectively.[5]

With TAA, documented complications can be categorized chronologically into intraoperative, postoperative, and late complications. Factors such as patient selection, surgeon experience, implant features, and prosthetic device selection can influence functional outcomes as well as incidence of complications. Even with impeccable surgical technique and optimal patient selection, complications that require revision may still arise and the most common complications with revision solutions are discussed in this article.

INDICATIONS

There are few outcome studies regarding revision surgery and there are a limited number of surgeons who have performed enough revisions to contribute to the literature. Consequently, indications for revision surgery are not well established. Factors that should be considered include the following: symptoms, pain, subsidence, alignment, bone stock, infection, and component integrity.[6] The most common early complications are ligament imbalance or component: malpositioning, subsidence, and/or impingement. Any of these situations may necessitate revision surgery to reduce the risk of premature TAA failure. Typically, late complications are due to wear of the polyethylene liner either from normal wear or from malalignment, aseptic loosening/osteolysis usually from polyethylene debris, or recurrent and or progressive frontal plane deformity. Early recognition of these complications will lessen the complexity of the revision surgery necessary to yield a functioning prosthesis.

When a failing or failed total ankle is encountered, a surgeon is faced with considering a complex revision arthroplasty versus salvage procedures that include the following: conversion to fusion, cement block interposition, and amputation.[7] With significant bone loss, conversion to arthrodesis is difficult because of loss of structural bone support and inability to place adequate fixation. This can be further complicated by nonunion and progressive arthritis of adjacent joints.[8–10] If standard components are not sufficient, a different prosthesis or larger components can be used in conjunction with bone graft.[7,8] Custom components also can be ordered to better fit the anatomic constraints of revision. Historically, custom components were ordered to better fit the anatomic constraints of revision. The authors have used many stemmed talar components in the past with excellent results in an otherwise very difficult revision. Manufacturers have decreased production of stemmed and custom components due to increased restrictions and more stringent Food and Drug Administration regulations. This has created a conundrum at best for patients that need revision. Surgeon creativity and need are blocked due to unavailability of these custom implants. Unfortunately, it is the patient in need of revision that has limited options due to these restrictions (**Box 1**).

Box 1
Complications of total ankle replacement

Intraoperative

- Dorsalis pedis laceration
- Posterior tibial artery laceration
- Component malalignment/incorrect sizing
- Malleolar fracture
- Nerve lacerations
- Posterior tibial tendon laceration
- Flexor digitorum longus tendon laceration
- Extensor hallucis longus tendon laceration
- Uncorrected deformity

Postoperative

- Component dislocation
- Component fracture
- Subsidence/aseptic loosening
- Fibular stress fracture
- Talar fracture
- Heterotopic bone formation
- Superficial or deep infection
- Ligamentous insufficiency/edge loading
- Complex regional pain syndrome
- Tarsal tunnel syndrome
- Incisional entrapment
- Syndesmotic nonunion (Agility)
- Osteolysis/lucencies
- Pain with stiffness
- Skin fistula
- Anterior tibial tendon necrosis
- Tendonitis
- Vascular compromise
- Venous embolic event
- Wound healing delay

Data from Schuberth JM, Steck, JK, Christensen, JC. Ankle replacement arthroplasty. In: Southerland JT, Boberg JS, Downey MS, et al, editors. Mcglamry's comprehensive textbook of foot and ankle surgery. 4th edition. Philadelphia: Wolters/Kluwer/Lippincott Williams & Wilkins Health; 2012. p. 743.

WOUND HEALING COMPLICATIONS

Dehiscence, incisional hematoma, and other wound healing complications are encountered in most clinical studies on TAA. The incidence of wound healing complications is highly variable in the literature but ranges from 4% to 28%.[11,12] The soft tissue envelope surrounding the ankle joint is thin, and previous surgery in the area can cause scarring and increase the risk for delayed healing.[13] The standard anterior incision lateral to tibialis anterior can disrupt the anterior tibial angiosome and choke vessels, increasing the risk for necrosis.[7,14] Other factors, such as aggressive soft tissue retraction, improper immobilization, immune suppression, and poor soft tissue envelope, can lead to complications and complication revisions. Diabetes mellitus is a known risk factor for wound healing complications in any surgery and is a risk factor in patients undergoing TAA.[11,14,15] A total of 32 of 220 total ankle replacements performed by the primary author between January 2011 and September 2016 were performed on patients with diabetes mellitus type 2. Overall incidence of wound healing complications in diabetic patients was 5 (15.6%) of 32.[16]

Dissection without delamination of layers, maintaining tibialis anterior in its sheath, careful handling of soft tissue, and layered wound closure are recommended. These wound healing issues are typically managed with parenteral antibiotics, local wound care, or negative-pressure wound therapy. Revision is often necessary in cases with full-thickness defects and larger wounds, and the patient may require a referral for plastic surgery for complex closure. It is paramount to treat wounds aggressively and promptly to prevent bacterial breach of the joint capsule that would lead to periprosthetic infection and need for major revision (**Figs. 1** and **2**).

DEEP PERIPROSTHETIC INFECTIONS

Deep periprosthetic infection (DPI) can lead to failure of TAA greater than 50% of the time.[1] In Gougoulias and colleagues,[17] systematic literature review of 827 total ankle replacements from 9 studies, the rate of deep infection ranged from 0% to 4.6%. Myerson and colleagues[18] reported a deep infection rate of 2.4% in their retrospective case series on 613 replacements. The authors' protocol for the diagnosis and treatment of periprosthetic ankle joint infections is adapted from the American Academy of Orthopedic Surgeons (AAOS) guidelines for the hip and knee[19] and literature from total knee arthroplasties.[19–21] Clinical suspicion is the most reliable element of the workup and unexplained total joint pain without obvious mechanical issues is secondary to infection until proven otherwise. Risk factors, such as immunocompromised status and other systemic symptoms of fever or malaise, for example, also increase suspicion. In their prospective study on 151 revision total knee arthroplasties in 145 patients, Greidanus and colleagues[21] determined that erythrocyte sedimentation rate (ESR) >22.5 mm/h and C-reactive protein (CRP) >13.5 mg/L is a reliable positive predictor of infection. Receiver-operating characteristic curve analysis was performed to determine optimal positivity criteria for each diagnostic test and compared with data using previously accepted established criteria (ESR $\geq$30 mm/h and CRP $\geq$10 mg/L) for infection after total hip arthroplasty.[22–24] Their established cutoff points correspond to the numerical threshold at which both sensitivity and the specificity of the test are optimized.

If both ESR and CRP are negative, infection is unlikely.[19] If ESR or CRP is elevated, it is recommended to aspirate the joint and send the fluid for microbiologic culture, synovial fluid white blood cell count, and differential.[19] In their review of 11,964 primary total knee arthroplasties (TKAs), Bedair and colleagues[20] identified 146 knees that had

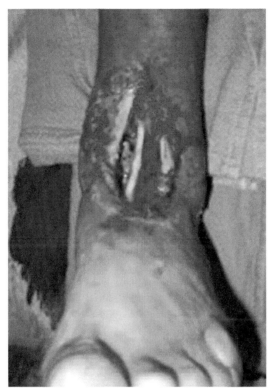

Fig. 1. Full-thickness necrosis of anterior incision with exposure of tibialis anterior and implant.

an aspiration within 6 weeks of surgery.[20] Their study showed synovial white blood cell count greater than 27,800 predicted infection within 6 weeks after primary TKA, with a positive predictive value of 94% and negative predictive value of 98%. If the joint aspirate is culture negative, it is recommended to repeat the joint aspiration.[19] Nuclear imaging (labeled leukocyte imaging) is indicated if the workup is negative but clinical suspicion remains or the patient is high risk.[19] Other technology is available, such as alpha defensin but is beyond the scope of this article, the reader is referred to the AAOS guidelines for further information.

If DPI is found, the implant is typically removed, antibiotic spacer placed, and a revision performed after clinical findings and infection markers have returned to normal. This is known as a 2-stage revision (**Figs. 3–11**). One-stage revisions in which the infected implant is removed and a new implant inserted in the same setting are much less common.

DPI also can be treated with conversion to fusion or by leaving the antibiotic spacer in place. Myerson and colleagues[18] reviewed 613 replacements and 7 of 19 cases of infection were treated with a permanent antibiotic spacer. Subluxation of cement was the only issue noted and is typically due to incorrect insertion.[18] Their treatment protocol consists of maximum distraction during insertion with a lamina spreader and ensuring the cement fills all voids.[18] DPIs are limb-threatening and life-threatening diagnoses; competent and emergent care should be delivered.

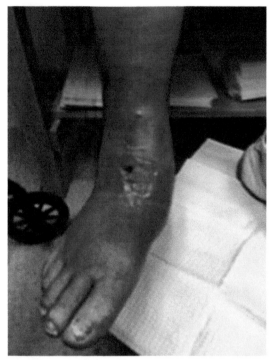

Fig. 2. Superficial dehiscence of anterior incision due to seroma.

JOINT STIFFNESS

Hip and knee arthroplasty typically start range of motion the day of surgery or at least postoperative day 1; this is not possible in TAA. Incision healing will just not allow early range of motion at the ankle, therefore scar tissue forms and ultimately range of motion

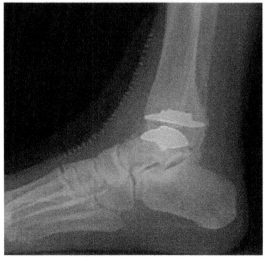

Fig. 3. Immediate postoperative TAA.

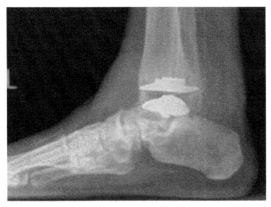

Fig. 4. Eight months postoperative.

is not as great. These facts inherently lead to issues and complaints regarding joint stiffness. Occasionally patients achieve greater range of motion than what they had before surgery.

Joint stiffness after total ankle arthroplasty is often multifactorial. Prior trauma and previous surgery can cause the thin soft tissue envelope to become scarred and stiff.[13] Prolonged immobilization, ineffective rehabilitation, poor soft tissue envelope, overstuffing the joint, inadequate soft tissue release, heterotopic bone growth, multiple operations, and previous infection can contribute to decreased range of

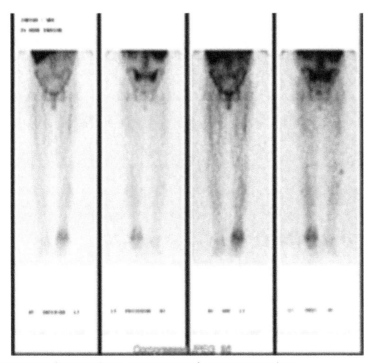

Fig. 5. Positive technetium bone scan 2 years after primary implant.

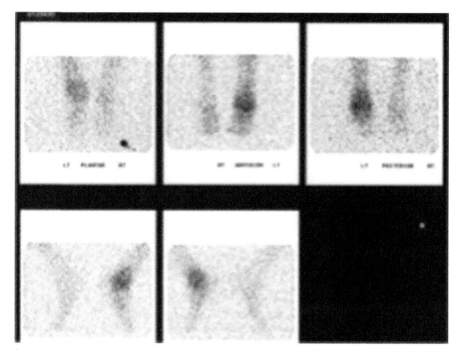

Fig. 6. Magnification of positive technetium bone scan 2 years after primary implant.

motion.[7,25] Intraoperatively, surgeon experience determines the optimal thickness of the implant components to maximize range of motion without sacrificing stability. Using a thinner polyethylene liner, removing osteophytes, and Achilles tendon lengthening or gastrocnemius recession can increase dorsiflexion.[25] A structured rehabilitation protocol and physical therapy are recommended to increase range of motion.

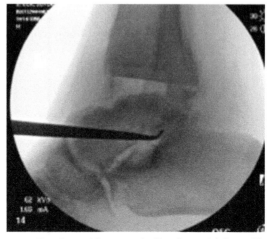

Fig. 7. Lateral intraoperative view with removal of implant with lateral bone loss from talus. Curette identifies significant loss of talar bone laterally.

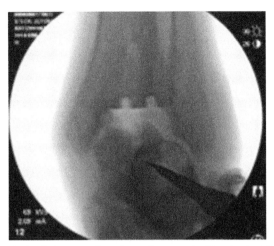

Fig. 8. Anterior posterior intraoperative view of removal of implant with lateral bone loss from talus.

There is no established uniform rehabilitation for TAA in the literature. Many times joint stiffness is not symptomatic or functionally detrimental to the patient if the arc of motion is in a functional range. If joint stiffness is symptomatic, and a specific reason can be found, such as inadequate Achilles tendon release, these can be addressed. Manipulation or debridement of scar tissue can help, although studies are unavailable on the outcome of these procedures, it is the authors' experience that they are minimally successful and need to be done very aggressively for best results.

The authors recommend non–weight bearing for at least 2 weeks until the incision has healed to decrease wound healing complications and to prevent shear forces on the components. The primary author's postoperative protocol requires non–weight bearing in a posterior plaster-of-Paris splint with the ankle at 90° for 2 weeks. The surgical incision is evaluated at 1 and 2 weeks and staples are typically removed at 2 weeks. The patient is then placed in a surgical boot and instructed to perform ankle

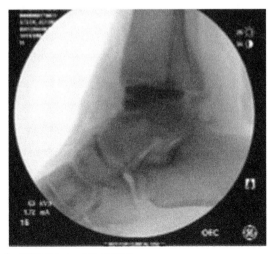

Fig. 9. Insertion of antibiotic cement spacer.

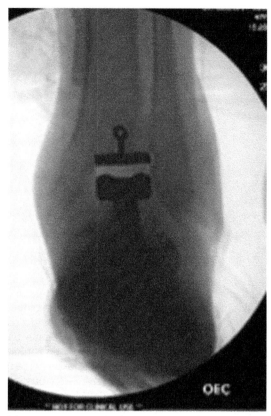

Fig. 10. Revision with custom stemmed talar component (anterior posterior view).

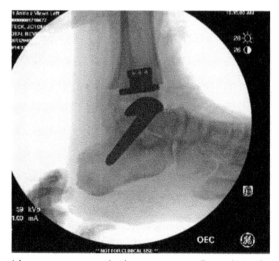

Fig. 11. Revision with custom stemmed talar component (lateral view).

range of motion exercises. At 6 weeks, the patient will wean out of the boot and begin aggressive physical therapy.

Mann and colleagues[26] reported on long-term survivorship of the STAR total ankle implant; 84 total ankle replacements were performed in 80 patients and followed prospectively. Postoperatively, patients were immobilized for 2 weeks and allowed to weight-bear in a cam-walker at 2 to 4 weeks.[26] Ninety-one percent of the prostheses remained implanted at an average follow-up of 9.1 years.[26]

PROSTHETIC MALALIGNMENT

In a normal ankle joint, the weight-bearing axis passes from the midline of the tibia to the heel, creating a valgus moment because it is slightly lateral to the ankle joint.[27,28] Likewise, in TAA, the weight-bearing axis should also have a valgus moment with the axis passing slightly lateral to the midline of the components.

One of the most common causes of alignment errors is due to misinterpretation of the tibial axis.[7] In our study of 50 total ankle replacements, we surmised that prosthetic malalignment could occur when there was insufficient intraoperative imaging of the tibial axis.[29] It is important to take into account the entire long axis of the leg intraoperatively, as constrained fluoroscopic imaging can skew alignment.[7,29] We also found that surgeon experience may influence component placement.[29] In the same study, we found the rate of major revision decreased 40% in their second cohort of 25 patients. We attributed this to increased appreciation of the tibial axis with experience. Proper component alignment is paramount to the success of ankle replacement, as tilting of the talar component can cause increased concentration of forces between the component-bone and polyethylene liner-component interfaces.[29] Increased poly wear should be expected if malalignment exists and is usually due to edge loading or shear forces.

If malalignment is found, it usually requires revision, as the imbalance is progressive and will lead to failure. Specific techniques are similar to those discussed in frontal plane deformities, as discussed later in this article. However, this can be monitored and braced if not symptomatic to a point; there are no standards or guidelines, which further underscores the importance of surgeon experience, as detailed in the discussion.

SUBSIDENCE

Subsidence is usually a late complication, and the process in which a component migrates deeper into osseous substrate.[7,30] Minor subsidence is expected postoperatively and typically decreases at 3 months. This process stabilizes at approximately 6 months. If component migration persists after 6 months, it is usually indicative of unstable bone-implant interfaces. On radiographs, component migration equal to or greater than 5 mm or 5° is considered unstable.[25] Talar component subsidence is more common than tibial component subsidence due to decreased peripheral cortical coverage. This can progress until the talar component violates the subtalar joint. Tibial component subsidence is infrequent and will occur more posteriorly with osseous lipping surrounding the posterior edge of the implant,[7] (**Figs. 12–14**). This is particularly true with implants that do not cover the posterior cortex of the tibia. Revision surgery for subsidence must include a workup of why the subsidence occurred in the first place, and the surgeon should be convinced that this will be corrected before or during surgery. With revision surgery, the joint line must be restored with a combination of bone graft, cement, and revision components that can replace the periarticular bone loss that is typically encountered. Limitations exist on revision components, as mentioned in the introduction, and polyethylene thicknesses are improved but limited

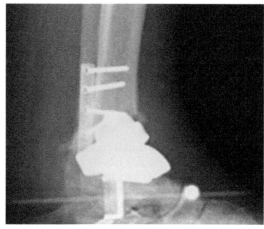

Fig. 12. Agility with anterior subsidence of tibial component and anterior subluxation.

as well. Therefore the surgeon is usually left to devise a plan consisting of bone graft and/or cement to make up for bone loss caused by subsidence (**Figs. 15–18**).

POLYETHYLENE WEAR AND ASEPTIC LOOSENING

Aseptic loosening is one major cause of decreased longevity in TAA, as well as all total joints, and can cause the implant to loosen prematurely.[7,31] It is defined as

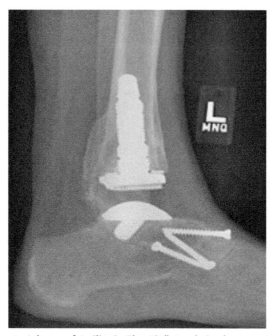

Fig. 13. Conversion to Inbone of Agility in **Fig. 12** (lateral view).

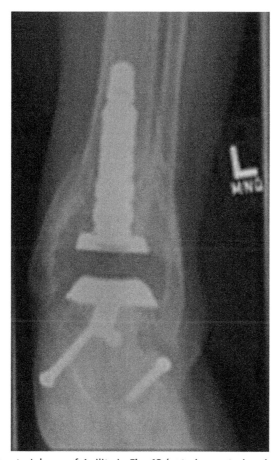

Fig. 14. Conversion to Inbone of Agility in **Fig. 12** (anterior posterior view).

bone loss that is not infectious and commonly used synonymously with osteolysis. The wear rate of polyethylene is influenced by multiple factors, including activity, quality and design of the insert, and placement.[7] In their study, Vaupel and colleagues[32] examined 10 failed Agility implants to determine wear patterns. Six patterns were noted on all polyethylene liners: burnishing, embedding, grooving/scratching, pitting, dishing, and abrasion.[32] The investigators called the area of the polyethylene liner with the most surface damage the "talar footprint," representing the area in which the talar component primarily articulated.[32] They also found titanium particles in the talar footprint of the retrieved liners demonstrating third body wear. This is the destructive wear of a prosthesis that involves particular matter that migrates along the articulating surface of the prosthetic components.[7] Kobayashi and colleagues[33] analyzed polyethylene particles from synovial fluid from 15 patients with total ankle arthroplasties and found them to be comparable to 11 patients with posterior stabilized TKAs at least 6 months postoperatively. Particulate polyethylene debris can incite a chronic inflammatory process that causes aseptic loosening.[34] The etiology again must be determined before revision. Diagnosis is predominantly done with plain radiographs and computed tomography

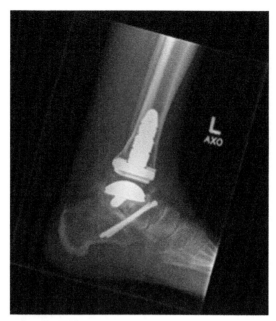

Fig. 15. Subsidence of talar component into subtalar joint.

(**Figs. 19** and **20**). Most ankle arthroplasties will develop at least a focal region of osteolysis, but whether this leads to aseptic loosening or not must be evaluated, and we recommend follow-up annually for surveillance radiographs. Goals of treatment are to restore bone stock, achieve stability, and correct if possible any cause

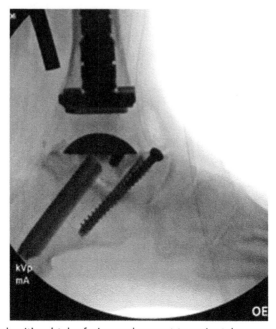

Fig. 16. Fusion rods with subtalar fusion and cement to revise talar component subsidence.

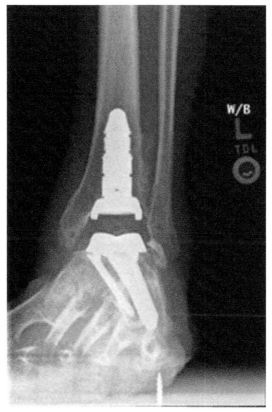

Fig. 17. Four years postoperative (anterior posterior view).

of poly wear (**Fig. 21**). If cysts are progressive, they must be cleaned out and filled with bone graft. Cement can be used for such defects but is much harder than bone and can stress shield; we prefer to use the impaction bone graft technique if possible. Often in symptomatic aseptic loosening, the implant needs to be removed and fresh cuts taken with bigger implants to fill up space from resected bone.

CYST FORMATION

Cyst formation is a common radiographic finding after TAA. Cysts can be a source of pain in patients who present with nonspecific symptoms. Small cysts often result from stress shielding around the implant.[6] Cyst formation along with pain and subsidence is a relative indication for revision.[6] Knecht and colleagues[3] defined lucencies as a radiolucent line ≤2 mm in width and lysis as a radiolucent area >2 mm. Lysis is further categorized as mechanical or expansile. Mechanical lysis is focal and occurs during the first 6 to 12 months and usually stabilizes.[3] Expansile lysis occurs later and is secondary to particle debris and an inflammatory process.[3] Expansile and mechanical lysis can be further categorized as stable or progressive and radiographs should be taken to monitor for acute changes.

When to intervene for enlarging cysts is ill defined. Clearly, intervention should be taken before pathologic fracture, which makes revision much more difficult. The

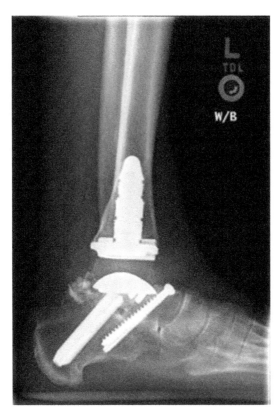

Fig. 18. Four years postoperative (lateral view).

authors use the flowchart in **Fig. 21**, as the algorithm is similar to treatment for aseptic loosening.

When intervention is undertaken, a window may need to be created to access the cyst, and the cyst is completely cleaned out to remove all irritants (usually poly debris) responsible for the inflammatory response (**Fig. 22**). This often resembles coffee grounds. Proximal tibial cancellous autograft is frequently used; it is easily accessible and typically provides adequate amounts of graft. Iliac crest is used if more volume is needed. Allograft or synthetic graft also can be used. Cement is not generally recommended, as it will cause stress shielding. A recent article reported findings with large cystic lesions in the Agility[35]; however, the investigators did not take into account the cause of the lesions and loosening, did not correct the reason for the loosening, and used Kirschner-wires in cement, which serves no added benefit to the (already stress shielding) strong cement. Furthermore, they used the same implant without changing its position, thus the biological process of osteolysis will continue and sentence the patient to continued osteolysis and future revision, making this technique very cost ineffective and ill conceived. The reader is cautioned against this technique as reported in our letter to the editor.[36]

FRONTAL PLANE DEFORMITY

If coronal plane deformity and ankle instability are not addressed primarily, there is increased incidence of loosening, failure, and polyethylene wear due to edge

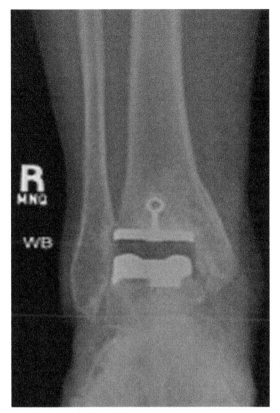

Fig. 19. Aseptic loosening surrounding tibial component.

loading.[25] In a study of 531 total ankle replacements, Henricson and colleagues[2] found 11 of 16 cases required revision for varus malalignment. In the study by Shock and colleagues[37] on primary TAA in the varus ankle, they described a step-wise surgical approach for varus deformity correction and compared the correction

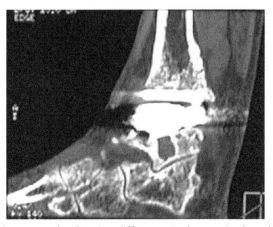

Fig. 20. Computed tomography showing diffuse cystic changes in the talus.

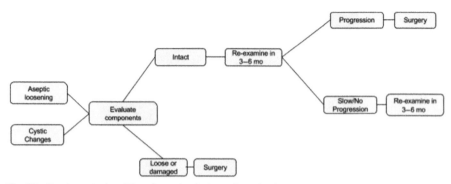

Fig. 21. Treatment algorithm for osteolysis and cystic changes.

of large frontal plane varus deformities using 2 different total ankle replacement systems. The retrospective study consisted of 26 patients, and all but 1 was corrected to within 4° of frontal plane neutral after primary TAA.[37] Revision for recurrent or newly developed frontal plane deformity parallels that of correction of frontal plane deformity correction before TAA. Usually 1 or more of the concepts were not addressed primarily. Although one can monitor frontal plane deformities with surveillance films, these are usually progressive and require treatment (**Figs. 23–25**). The sequence of corrective maneuvers for varus deformities is described in **Box 2**.

CONTRAINDICATIONS

Absolute contraindications to revisional arthroplasty include active infection, poor soft tissue envelope, insufficient bone stock, inability to heal, and Charcot

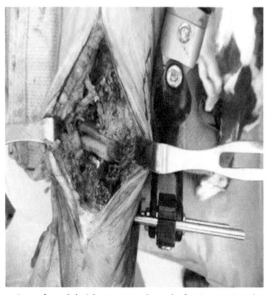

Fig. 22. Cystic formation after debridement and ready for impaction bone grafting.

neuroarthropathy. Patients who have had prior revisions, extensive bone loss, history of infection, and previous wound healing complications are at higher risk of developing complications.[7] Patients who are not good candidates for TAA revision may require bracing with an ankle-foot orthosis.

DISCUSSION

Complications in TAA can be severe; in fact, periprosthetic joint infections are life-threatening and rival mortality of carotid surgery, kidney transplantation, and even coronary intervention (**Fig. 26**).[38] It cannot be expressed enough that proper training be established before taking on these difficult cases. Avoiding complications is clearly preferable; the learning curve that accompanies TAA is high and has been a criticism of TAA since its inception, yet it is real and must be managed and controlled. Many of the learning curve complications can be avoided in most cases by proper education, training, and experience.

TAA requires the unique skill-set of a total joint, as well as a reconstructive foot and ankle surgeon. Most pure total joint surgeons do not have the foot and ankle experience needed to address or even recognize alignment issues in the foot and leg; whereas, most reconstructive foot and ankle surgeons lack the focused education, training, and experience to effectively execute a safe and efficient total joint surgery.

When initially performing TAA, surgeons encounter a steep learning curve that inherently leads to complications that are mostly preventable.[29,39] However, with focused training by experienced TAA surgeons, surgeons in training subsequently have a significantly lower rate of complications.[40] Surgeon experience and volume also contribute to overall reduced complications. In a cohort of 4800 TAA cases performed by 1808 surgeons; high-volume surgeons (more than 21 cases per year) had a 42.9% lower complication rate when compared with low-volume surgeons (fewer than 21 cases per year).[41] This study revealed that 53% of the TAA surgeon pool performed 5 or fewer cases per year.[41] Thus, many surgeons

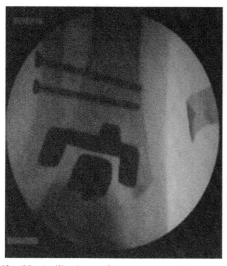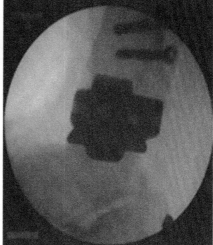

Fig. 23. Agility immediate postoperative.

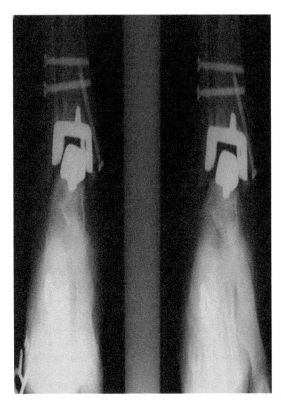

Fig. 24. Postoperative medial malleolar fracture due to progression of valgus deformity.

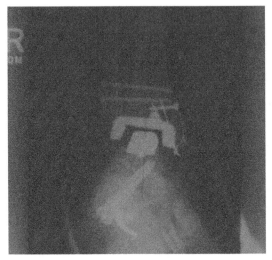

Fig. 25. Eight months postoperative repair of recurrent medial malleolar fracture and subtalar fusion. This case highlights the importance of correcting deformity initially as these are progressive and will cause failure if not corrected.

Box 2
Sequence of varus deformity correction
Ancillary pedal procedures
Standard incisional approach
Medial deltoid sleeve release
Lateral gutter resection to allow lateral displacement and derotation of the talus
Talar deformity reduction
Tibial-talar preparation
Insertion of components
Lateral ligament plication
Data from Shock RP, Christensen JC, Schuberth JM. Total ankle replacement in the varus ankle. J Foot Ankle Surg 2011;50(1):5–10.

performing TAA may be ill-equipped to execute a revision strategy because of their low-volume experience.

Prophylactic measures help to reduce the impact of complexity of revision via early identification of the problem. We recommend annual surveillance of every total ankle placed in each practice. It is a given that a certain percentage of cases will need revision

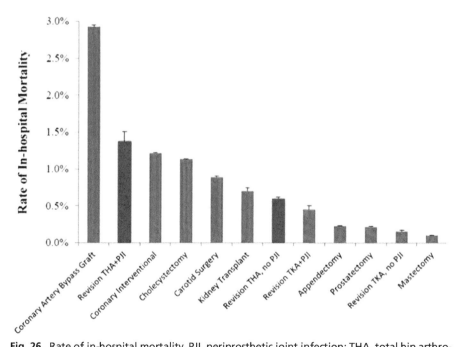

Fig. 26. Rate of in-hospital mortality. PJI, periprosthetic joint infection; THA, total hip arthroplasty. (*Data from* Shahi A, Tan T, Chen A, et al. In-hospital morality in patients with periprosthetic joint infection. Poster presented at: AAOS 2016 Annual Meeting. Orlando (FL), March 1–5, 2016.)

at some point. The key with surveillance is to preemptively identify the individuals that may need revision and closely monitor and educate these patients. It is much easier to intervene early and revise the implant before it has reached a point in which the prosthesis has completely failed. Patients who are having functional difficulties tend to appreciate a surgeon's interest in close monitoring of their condition. In some cases, there may be activities that are aggravating the function of the implant (ie, heavy lifting, repetitive stress at work) that can be modified to improve prosthesis function and longevity.

In our experience, there are joints that are being revised unnecessarily due to lack of understanding, experience, and recognition of the natural course of TAA. In some cases, there are revisable joints that are unnecessarily being converted to fusion. Hopefully in the future, criteria can be developed to form rational clinical pathways for surgeons considering revision TAA.

SUMMARY

TAA is a difficult procedure with a high learning curve. Revision TAA is even more demanding and requires experienced surgeons to undertake. Many of the principles for revision are the same no matter what the cause that created the need for revision. These principles are as follows:

- Ensure infection is eradicated
- Ensure alignment
- Fill resultant defect with a combination of implant, bone graft, and cement to provide stability to revisional implant
- Correct cause of failure

REFERENCES

1. Glazebrook MA, Arsenault K, Dunbar M. Evidence-based classification of complications in total ankle arthroplasty. Foot Ankle Int 2009;30(10):945–9.
2. Henricson A, Carlsson A, Rydholm U. What is a revision of total ankle replacement? Foot Ankle Surg 2011;17(3):99–102.
3. Knecht SI, Estin M, Callaghan JJ, et al. The Agility total ankle arthroplasty. Seven to sixteen-year follow-up. J Bone Joint Surg Am 2004;86A(6):1161–71.
4. Daniels TR, Younger AS, Penner M, et al. Intermediate-term results of total ankle replacement and ankle arthrodesis: a COFAS multicenter study. J Bone Joint Surg Am 2014;96(2):135–42.
5. Steck JK, Anderson JB. Total ankle arthroplasty: indications and avoiding complications. Clin Podiatr Med Surg 2009;26(2):303–24.
6. Meeker J, Wegner N, Francisco R, et al. Revision techniques in total ankle arthroplasty utilizing a stemmed tibial arthroplasty system. Tech Foot Ankle Surg 2013; 12(2):99–108.
7. Schuberth JM, Steck JK, Christensen JC. Ankle replacement arthroplasty. In: Southerland JT, Boberg JS, Downey MS, et al, editors. Mcglamry's comprehensive textbook of foot and ankle surgery. 4th edition. Philadelphia: Wolters/Kluwer/Lippincott Williams & Wilkins Health; 2012. p. 717–56.
8. Myerson MS, Won HY. Primary and revision total ankle replacement using custom-designed prostheses. Foot Ankle Clin 2008;13(3):521–38, x.
9. Haddad SL, Coetzee JC, Estok R, et al. Intermediate and long-term outcomes of total ankle arthroplasty and ankle arthrodesis. A systematic review of the literature. J Bone Joint Surg Am 2007;89(9):1899–905. Review.

10. Haskell A, Mann RA. Perioperative complication rate of total ankle replacement is reduced by surgeon experience. Foot Ankle Int 2004;25(5):283–9.
11. Whalen JL, Spelsberg SC, Murray P. Wound breakdown after total ankle arthroplasty. Foot Ankle Int 2010;31(4):301–5.
12. Farber DC, Deorio JK. Oxygen tensiometry as a predictor of wound healing in total ankle arthroplasty. Acta Orthop Traumatol Turc 2009;43(5):381–5.
13. Conti SF, Wong YS. Complications of total ankle replacement. Foot Ankle Clin 2002;7(4):791–807, vii. Review.
14. Raikin SM, Kane J, Ciminiello ME. Risk factors for incision-healing complications following total ankle arthroplasty. J Bone Joint Surg Am 2010;92(12):2150–5.
15. Choi WJ, Lee JS, Lee M, et al. The impact of diabetes on the short- to mid-term outcome of total ankle replacement. Bone Joint J 2014;96B(12):1674–80.
16. Luu CA, Steck JK. Wound healing complications in diabetics after total ankle replacement. Poster presented at: Desert Foot Conference. Phoenix (AZ), October 19–21, 2016.
17. Gougoulias N, Khanna A, Maffulli N. How successful are current ankle replacements? Clin Orthop Relat Res 2010;469:199–208.
18. Myerson MS, Shariff R, Zonno AJ. The management of infection following total ankle replacement: demographics and treatment. Foot Ankle Int 2014;35(9): 855–62.
19. Parvizi J, Della Valle CJ. AAOS Clinical Practice Guideline: diagnosis and treatment of periprosthetic joint infections of the hip and knee. J Am Acad Orthop Surg 2010;18(12):771–2.
20. Bedair H, Ting N, Jacovides C, et al. The Mark Coventry Award: diagnosis of early postoperative TKA infection using synovial fluid analysis. Clin Orthop Relat Res 2011;469(1):34–40.
21. Greidanus NV, Masri BA, Garbuz DS, et al. Use of erythrocyte sedimentation rate and C-reactive protein level to diagnose infection before revision total knee arthroplasty. A prospective evaluation. J Bone Joint Surg Am 2007;89(7):1409–16.
22. Spangehl MJ, Masri BA, O'Connell JX, et al. Prospective analysis of preoperative and intraoperative investigations for the diagnosis of infection at the sites of two hundred and two revision total hip arthroplasties. J Bone Joint Surg Am 1999;81: 672–83.
23. Niskanen RO, Korkala O, Pammo H. Serum C-reactive protein levels after total hip and knee arthroplasty. J Bone Joint Surg Br 1996;78:431–3.
24. White J, Kelly M, Dunsmuir R. C-reactive protein level after total hip and total knee replacement. J Bone Joint Surg Br 1998;80:909–11.
25. Jonck JH, Myerson MS. Revision total ankle replacement. Foot Ankle Clin 2012; 17(4):687–706.
26. Mann JA, Mann RA, Horton E. STAR™ ankle: long-term results. Foot Ankle Int 2011;32(5):S473–84.
27. Greisberg J, Hansen ST Jr. Ankle replacement: management of associated deformities. Foot Ankle Clin 2002;7(4):721–36, vi.
28. Harrington KD. Degenerative arthritis of the ankle secondary to long-standing lateral ligament instability. J Bone Joint Surg 1979;61A:354–61.
29. Schuberth JM, Patel S, Zarutsky E. Perioperative complications of the Agility total ankle replacement in 50 initial, consecutive cases. J Foot Ankle Surg 2006;45(3): 139–46.
30. Pyevich MT, Saltzman CL, Callaghan JJ, et al. Total ankle arthroplasty: a unique design. Two to twelve-year follow-up. J Bone Joint Surg Am 1998;80(10): 1410–20.

31. Espinosa N, Walti M, Favre P, et al. Misalignment of total ankle components can induce high joint contact pressures. J Bone Joint Surg Am 2010;92(5):1179–87.

32. Vaupel Z, Baker EA, Baker KC, et al. Analysis of retrieved agility total ankle arthroplasty systems. Foot Ankle Int 2009;30(9):815–23.

33. Kobayashi A, Minoda Y, Kadoya Y, et al. Ankle arthroplasties generate wear particles similar to knee arthroplasties. Clin Orthop Relat Res 2004;(424):69–72.

34. Gill LH. Challenges in total ankle arthroplasty. Foot Ankle Int 2004;25(4):195–207.

35. Prissel MA, Roukis TS. Management of extensive tibial osteolysis with the Agility™ total ankle replacement systems using geometric metal-reinforced polymethylmethacrylate cement augmentation. J Foot Ankle Surg 2014;53(1):101–7.

36. Schuberth JM, Steck JK, Christensen JC. Ill-conceived total ankle revision technique. J Foot Ankle Surg 2014;53(3):390–1.

37. Shock RP, Christensen JC, Schuberth JM. Total ankle replacement in the varus ankle. J Foot Ankle Surg 2011;50(1):5–10.

38. Shahi A, Tan T, Chen A, et al. In-hospital morality in patients with periprosthetic joint infection. Poster presented at: AAOS 2016 Annual Meeting. Orlando (FL), March 1–5, 2016.

39. Myerson MS, Mroczek K. Perioperative complications of total ankle arthroplasty. Foot Ankle Int 2003;24(1):17–21.

40. Saltzman CL, Mann RA, Ahrens JE, et al. Prospective controlled trial of STAR total ankle replacement versus ankle fusion: initial results. Foot Ankle Int 2009;30(7):579–96.

41. Basques BA, Bitterman A, Campbell KJ, et al. Influence of surgeon volume on inpatient complications, cost, and length of stay following total ankle arthroplasty. Foot Ankle Int 2016;37:1046–51.

Surgical Complications of Ankle Joint Arthrodesis and Ankle Arthroplasty Procedures

 CrossMark

Benjamin D. Overley Jr, DPM[a],*, Matthew R. Rementer, DPM[b]

KEYWORDS

• Total ankle arthroplasty • Ankle arthrodesis • Complications • Infection

KEY POINTS

• Complications are a very real risk when dealing with total ankle arthroplasty (TAA) and ankle arthrodesis (AA) that the physician must be ready to handle before undertaking the initial surgery.
• The most common complications in TAA are deep infection and implant failure when looking at the short-term and long-term.
• The most common complications in AA are nonunion and wound healing complications.
• Recent literature has shown a decrease in complications after TAA and AA surgeries.

INTRODUCTION

When looking at all surgeries, one of the most important things that must always be considered are the complications. Surgeons must be prepared to handle the complications of the surgery before under taking it. When looking at total ankle arthroplasty (TAA) and ankle arthrodesis (AA), we are looking at very serious complications that could lead to limb loss. The two surgeries have some very similar complications along with some that are very different. The most common minor complication seen in both surgeries is wound healing complications ranging from 1% to 6%[1–3] (**Fig. 1**). The most common major complication for AA is nonunion of the fusion site.[2–4] This complication is usually seen in about 2% to 10% of ankle fusion surgery but is possibly decreased with new techniques in AA surgery.[4] When looking at TAA, the most common major complication is deep infection, ranging in about 3% to 10% of surgeries when looking at the short-term.[5] When looking at the long-term, the most common major

Disclosure Statement: Wright Medical Group, Amniox Medical, Inc.
[a] Foot and Ankle Surgery, Coventry Foot and Ankle Surgery, 296 W. Ridge Pike, Limerick, PA 19468, USA; [b] Podiatric Medicine and Surgery Residency, Phoenixville Hospital, 140 Nutt Road, Phoenixville, PA 19460, USA
* Corresponding author.
E-mail address: benjamin.overley@gmail.com

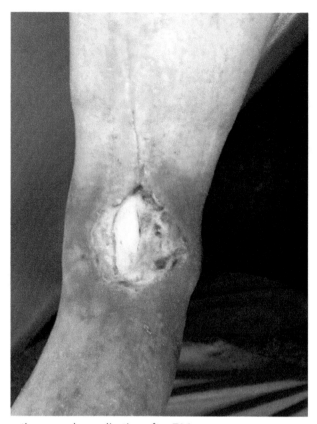

Fig. 1. Postoperative wound complication after TAA.

complication of TAA is implant failure in 5% to 15%.[6] It has been noted that with new advances in both surgeries, there has been a decrease in complication rates over the past 10 years.[2,7,8] Although, with both surgeries, especially TAA, a learning curve is noted with higher risk of complications for surgeons with less experience.[2] The most common complications seen with TAA are implant failure, aseptic loosening/subsidence, osteolysis, polyethylene liner fracture, hardware pain, nerve injury, malalignment, heterotopic ossification, wound problems, infection, perioperative fractures, deep vein thrombosis (DVT), adjacent joint arthritis, and amputation[1] (**Fig. 2**). The most common complications seen with AA are hardware pain, hardware failure, nonunion, malunion, wound problems, nerve injury, infection, perioperative fractures, DVT, adjacent joint arthritis, and amputation[1] (**Fig. 3**). The key to handling the complications of both surgeries is early recognition and treatment.

PATIENT EVALUATION OVERVIEW

With all situations in medicine, the most important aspect of evaluating patients is a thorough history and physical examination. This comprehensive approach point is especially true for examining patients postoperatively when looking for complications. This evaluation begins at the first postoperative visit when looking for signs and symptoms for infection including systemic symptoms and local symptoms. As the postoperative course continues, the physician must continue to keep a close eye out for any

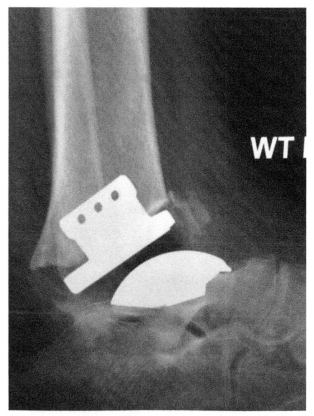

Fig. 2. Implant failure due to cystic changes in the bone that were not noted preoperatively.

abnormalities that may be a sign of a complication. Calf pain or redness or warmth must be evaluated for possible DVT in all cases through a venous ultrasound Doppler. If this is identified, it must be appropriately identified. The next step in evaluation would be radiographic examinations. These examinations include your standard radiographs followed by your more in-depth studies, including computed tomography (CT) scan, single-photon emission CT (SPECT)-CT scan, 3-phase bone scan, and in some cases MRI. Radiographs are an excellent starting point to evaluate the ankle but do not always show you the entire story. When evaluating for fusion, a CT scan will allow for a better understanding of how much of the joint is fused. It can also be a helpful tool in assessing the position of the components of the TAA. CT scans also allow you to note cystic changes in the bone that may be causing changes in the positioning of the components. Another excellent tool in assessing the implants and their failure is an SPECT-CT scan (**Fig. 4**). This scan allows for excellent visualization of the implants and their subsidence. Three-phase bone scan is a classic way to look for infection around the implant that still has its place today in evaluating for periprosthetic infections. This can be taken one step further with white blood cell–labeled bone scans. Finally, MRI may be used in certain situations to evaluate for soft tissue infection when the hardware is MRI compatible. Next, your standard blood tests are still useful in evaluating for infection and inflammation. Complete blood count allows you to evaluate for infection, whereas an erythrocyte sedimentation rate and C-reactive protein

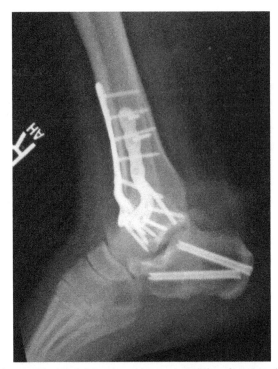

Fig. 3. Successful AA with painful hardware several months after noted fusion. Note the slightly plantigrade appearance at the ankle arthrodesis site.

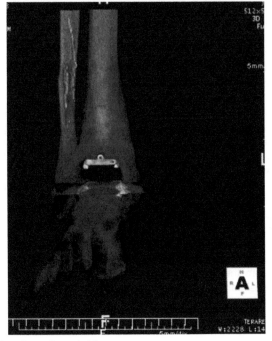

Fig. 4. SPECT-CT showing talar subsidence.

allow for evaluation of inflammation. Finally, if suspected, especially in a TAA, a joint aspirate can be performed to evaluate for infection or inflammation. This procedure must be done under sterile conditions to assure that you do not track bacteria into the joint.

PHARMACOLOGIC TREATMENT OPTIONS

The pharmacologic treatment options specifically pertain what complication that you are dealing with. When it comes to continued pain following TAA and AA, the treatment options consist of nonsteroidal antiinflammatory drugs (NSAIDs) and narcotics. The dosage and type of narcotic prescribed should be tailored to the patient, their activity level, and prior history of narcotic medication exposure. Pain management consultation may be needed in some of these patients, especially if this is going to be a long-term treatment option. In most of these situations, long-term NSAIDs are the better option versus short-term courses. These medications include meloxicam and others that work to suppress the inflammation on a long-term basis.

The largest pharmacologic treatment option resolves around one specific complication: infection. When dealing with superficial skin infections, the most common causative agents are *Staphylococcus* and *Streptococcus*. To treat these, the best course is usually a cephalosporin, such as cephalexin. It is important to identify risk factors that may put patients at risk for different bacteria. Methicillin-resistant *Staphylococcus aureus* exposure in the past is important to be identified as this may be causing the infection and must be covered in your antibiotic selection. Also, if patients are diabetic, they may be at risk for other unusual infective agents. It is important to always culture the wounds when possible so that you are assured of proper antibiotic coverage. When it comes to deeper infections, cultures should always be obtained to determine the proper antibiotics. The literature has not shown what is the best course for treating periprosthetic joint infections. The current literature suggests 2 to 6 weeks of intravenous (IV) antibiotics for the treatment of these infections. The standard of 6 weeks of IV antibiotics still exists for the treatment of all bone infections. The most common cause of deep infection in total joints and hardware is *Staphylococcus epidermidis*, but cultures to determine the causative bacteria are always necessary.

NONPHARMACOLOGIC TREATMENT OPTIONS

Again, the treatment of complications after TAA and AA that are nonpharmacologic varies depending on the specific complication. The most common complication in AA is nonunion, which has many different nonsurgical therapies. Bracing is one of the most common treatment options for both TAA and AA. Braces allow for patients with complications from TAA and AA to ambulate without pain as they restrict motion. For wound complications, standard wound healing techniques should be used. If these fail, use of grafts can be used to treat these patients. Grafting sources may include allograft, autograft such as block, particulate, or both or vascularized free grafts from alternative sites. The grafting may also be augmented with native bone marrow aspirate from the calcaneus, distal tibia, or ipsilateral anterior superior iliac crest if simultaneous bone harvesting from the hip is being contemplated. Specific to nonunion, bone stimulators are an excellent option to help increase bone activity at the fusion site with hopes to stimulate bone turnover allowing for further fusion. Several studies have shown an increase in healing with the use of bone stimulators in both fractures and fusions.

COMBINATION THERAPIES

Again, when it comes to conservative therapies for complications of TAA and AA, it is important to look at the specific needs of patients. When awaiting reimplantation for deep infection, a combination of antibiotics and bracing can be used for optimal therapy during this period of time. Also, bracing and pain medications can be used to control symptoms when the patient is not a surgical revision candidate. Most nonsurgical therapies when dealing with complications of TAA and AA are to hold patients until definitive surgical intervention is possible.

SURGICAL TREATMENT OPTIONS

For most complications following TAA and AA surgery, secondary surgeries are necessary. The additional surgeries that are required should be specific to the complication at hand. Starting with implant failure, revision surgery is often necessary. These surgeries can be combination rebuilds requiring talar, tibial, and poly components to be revised. For example, a revisional TAA may be more desirous to patients than converting a TAA to an AA, which can be challenging because of the inherent bone loss from the implant itself. TAA failure can be due to component subsidence (**Fig. 5**) or improper placement of the implant in the index procedure (**Fig. 6**). If heterotopic ossification is noted, surgery for debridement and removal of all bony growth is necessary to allow for full range of motion of the joint (**Fig. 7**). If fractures are noted both intraoperatively or postoperatively, open reduction with internal fixation may be necessary depending on the severity and the impact it can have on the survivorship of the implant. Polyethylene fracture or wear can be treated simply through polyethylene exchange. In cases whereby malalignment occurs, secondary procedures may be necessary to correct the deformities that are driving the malalignment (**Fig. 8**). In

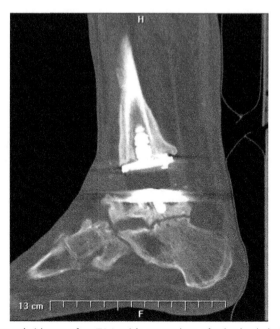

Fig. 5. Severe talar subsidence after TAA with severe loss of talar body height.

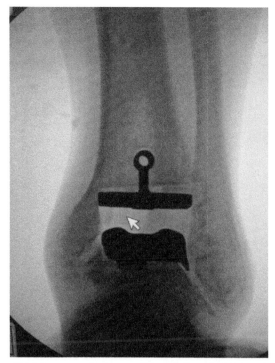

Fig. 6. Aggressive, tibial bone corticotomy with malaligned tibial and talar implantation and inadequate medial and lateral gutter debridement.

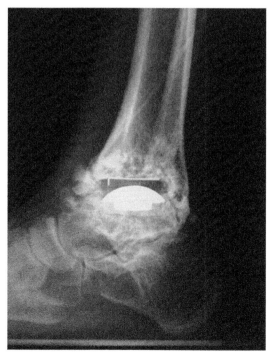

Fig. 7. Severe heterotopic ossification after TAA restricting motion.

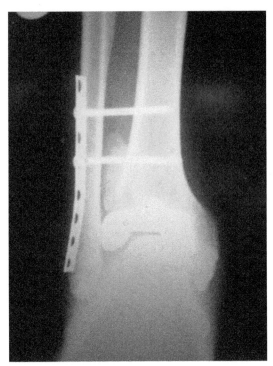

Fig. 8. Failed distal synostosis resulting in an unstable total ankle replacement.

some cases after TAA, adjacent joints may have preexisting arthritis that needs to be treated through arthrodesis of those joints. The most severe complication following TAA is deep infection. This complication must be immediately addressed surgically. Incision and debridement with extensive irrigation is the first stage of surgical treatment in deeply infected implants. Depending on the extent of the infection, removal of the implant may be necessary with implantation of an antibiotic cement spacer until clearance of the infection is noted. Once the infection is noted to be cleared, revisional surgery can be undertaken in the form of either revisional TAA or conversion to AA. In severe cases when osteomyelitis is present, amputation may be required.

When looking at the complications of AA, the surgical intervention necessary is much different compared with TAA. For nonunion or malunion, revision AA with autologous grafting and bone marrow aspirate to increase the likelihood of a bony union at the fusion site is often required. In cases whereby hardware pain exists, if the fusion is noted to be stable, removal of the hardware is an easy solution to this complication. One of the most common long-term complications of AA is adjacent joint arthritis. These adjacent joints typically will show early presence of arthritis before the AA being performed, and this process will rapidly accelerate once the ankle is formally fused. If these joints fail conservative treatments, arthrodesis of these joints may be needed. This complication is more common after AA compared with TAA. The treatment of deep infection in AA is very similar to the surgical treatment of TAA. Thorough irrigation and debridement is necessary immediately. Again, once the infection is noted to be completely eradicated, revision of the AA can be undertaken. In situations whereby bone infection is noted that cannot be removed, below-the-knee amputation may be necessary.

TREATMENT RESISTANCE/COMPLICATIONS

When managing postoperative complications in both TAA and AA, there is always the risk of resistance to treatment. This resistance may end in uncontrollable pain that is required to be managed by a pain specialist. As discussed earlier, the largest complication or failure to respond to therapy is amputation of the affected limb. These patients are already high risk after failure of the original surgery, which leads to increased chances for failure. It is important to discuss the very real chance of limb loss with patients who are undergoing secondary procedures because of complications, especially infection.

EVALUATION OF OUTCOME AND LONG-TERM RECOMMENDATIONS

As with all surgeries, outcomes are measured by patient satisfaction and postoperative pain and ability. When looking at TAA, the motion that is obtained at the ankle joint and function of patients is the most important outcome. For AA, propulsive gait that is pain free is the outcome that is most acceptable. After complications, the expected outcomes are less compared with patients who undergo the same surgery but do not have complications. For long-term management of these patients, close follow-up is needed to assure no reoccurrence of complications are noted. These patients are at higher risk for other complications.

SUMMARY/DISCUSSION

Complications of TAA and AA are very serious and can be life altering. Early identification of the complications is the most important aspect of treating these issues. When discussing these surgeries and consenting patients, it is imperative to have a long discussion of the risks and complications so that they fully understand what they are getting into. The complications should be taken very seriously, and understanding how to treat these is imperative before performing the initial surgery. In recent years, a decrease in complications has been noted in both surgeries. Although complications only occur in a small percentage of patients, it is important to be prepared for such issues.

REFERENCES

1. Kim HJ, Suh DH, Yang JH, et al. Total ankle arthroplasty versus ankle arthrodesis for the treatment of end-stage ankle arthritis: a meta-analysis of comparative studies. Int Orthop 2017;41(1):101–9.
2. Stavrakis AI, Soohoo NF. Trends in complication rates following ankle arthrodesis and total ankle replacement. J Bone Joint Surg Am 2016;98(17):1453–8.
3. SooHoo NF, Zingmond DS, Ko CY. Comparison of reoperation rates following ankle arthrodesis and total ankle arthroplasty. J Bone Joint Surg Am 2007;89(10):2143–9.
4. Townshend D, Di silvestro M, Krause F, et al. Arthroscopic versus open ankle arthrodesis: a multicenter comparative case series. J Bone Joint Surg Am 2013;95(2):98–102.
5. Gadd RJ, Barwick TW, Paling E, et al. Assessment of a three-grade classification of complications in total ankle replacement. Foot Ankle Int 2014;35(5):434–7.
6. Haddad SL, Coetzee JC, Estok R, et al. Intermediate and long-term outcomes of total ankle arthroplasty and ankle arthrodesis. A systematic review of the literature. J Bone Joint Surg Am 2007;89:1899–905.

7. Fevang B, Lie S, Havelin S, et al. 257 Ankle arthroplasties performed in Norway between 1994 and 2005. Acta Orthop 2007;78(5):575–83.

8. National Joint Registry for England and Wales. 9th Annual Report. Surgical data to 31st December 2011. 2012. Available at: http://www.njrcentre.org.uk/njrcentre/Portals/0/Documents/England/Reports/9th_annual_report/NJR%209th%20Annual%20Report%202012.pdf.

UNITED STATES POSTAL SERVICE®
Statement of Ownership, Management, and Circulation
(All Periodicals Publications Except Requester Publications)

1. Publication Title	2. Publication Number	3. Filing Date
CLINICS IN PODIATRIC MEDICINE & SURGERY	000 – 707	9/18/2017

4. Issue Frequency	5. Number of Issues Published Annually	6. Annual Subscription Price
JAN, APR, JUL, OCT	4	$288.00

7. Complete Mailing Address of Known Office of Publication (Not printer) (Street, city, county, state, and ZIP+4®)

ELSEVIER INC.
230 Park Avenue, Suite 800
New York, NY 10169

Contact Person: STEPHEN R. BUSHING
Telephone (Include area code): 215-239-3688

8. Complete Mailing Address of Headquarters or General Business Office of Publisher (Not printer)

ELSEVIER INC.
230 Park Avenue, Suite 800
New York, NY 10169

9. Full Names and Complete Mailing Addresses of Publisher, Editor, and Managing Editor (Do not leave blank)

Publisher (Name and complete mailing address)

ADRIANNE BRIGIDO, ELSEVIER INC.
1600 JOHN F KENNEDY BLVD. SUITE 1800
PHILADELPHIA, PA 19103-2899

Editor (Name and complete mailing address)

LAUREN BOYLE, ELSEVIER INC.
1600 JOHN F KENNEDY BLVD. SUITE 1800
PHILADELPHIA, PA 19103-2899

Managing Editor (Name and complete mailing address)

PATRICK MANLEY, ELSEVIER INC.
1600 JOHN F KENNEDY BLVD. SUITE 1800
PHILADELPHIA, PA 19103-2899

10. Owner (Do not leave blank. If the publication is owned by a corporation, give the name and address of the corporation immediately followed by the names and addresses of all stockholders owning or holding 1 percent or more of the total amount of stock. If not owned by a corporation, give the names and addresses of the individual owners. If owned by a partnership or other unincorporated firm, give its name and address as well as those of each individual owner. If the publication is published by a nonprofit organization, give its name and address.)

Full Name	Complete Mailing Address
WHOLLY OWNED SUBSIDIARY OF REED/ELSEVIER, US HOLDINGS	1600 JOHN F KENNEDY BLVD. SUITE 1800 PHILADELPHIA, PA 19103-2899

11. Known Bondholders, Mortgagees, and Other Security Holders Owning or Holding 1 Percent or More of Total Amount of Bonds, Mortgages, or Other Securities. If none, check box ▶ ☐ None

Full Name	Complete Mailing Address
N/A	

12. Tax Status (For completion by nonprofit organizations authorized to mail at nonprofit rates) (Check one)
The purpose, function, and nonprofit status of this organization and the exempt status for federal income tax purposes:
☒ Has Not Changed During Preceding 12 Months
☐ Has Changed During Preceding 12 Months (Publisher must submit explanation of change with this statement)

13. Publication Title	14. Issue Date for Circulation Data Below
CLINICS IN PODIATRIC MEDICINE & SURGERY	JULY 2017

15. Extent and Nature of Circulation		Average No. Copies Each Issue During Preceding 12 Months	No. Copies of Single Issue Published Nearest to Filing Date
a. Total Number of Copies (Net press run)		307	263
b. Paid Circulation (By Mail and Outside the Mail)	(1) Mailed Outside-County Paid Subscriptions Stated on PS Form 3541 (include paid distribution above nominal rate, advertiser's proof copies, and exchange copies)	182	167
	(2) Mailed In-County Paid Subscriptions Stated on PS Form 3541 (include paid distribution above nominal rate, advertiser's proof copies, and exchange copies)	0	0
	(3) Paid Distribution Outside the Mails Including Sales Through Dealers and Carriers, Street Vendors, Counter Sales, and Other Paid Distribution Outside USPS®	20	22
	(4) Paid Distribution by Other Classes of Mail Through the USPS (e.g. First-Class Mail®)	0	0
c. Total Paid Distribution (Sum of 15b (1), (2), (3), and (4))		202	189
d. Free or Nominal Rate Distribution (By Mail and Outside the Mail)	(1) Free or Nominal Rate Outside-County Copies included on PS Form 3541	71	74
	(2) Free or Nominal Rate In-County Copies Included on PS Form 3541	0	0
	(3) Free or Nominal Rate Copies Mailed at Other Classes Through the USPS (e.g. First-Class Mail)	0	0
	(4) Free or Nominal Rate Distribution Outside the Mail (Carriers or other means)	0	0
e. Total Free or Nominal Rate Distribution (Sum of 15d (1), (2), (3) and (4))		71	74
f. Total Distribution (Sum of 15c and 15e)		273	263
g. Copies not Distributed (See Instructions to Publishers #4 (page 43))		34	0
h. Total (Sum of 15f and g)		307	263
i. Percent Paid (15c divided by 15f times 100)		73.99%	71.86%

* If you are claiming electronic copies, go to line 16 on page 3. If you are not claiming electronic copies, skip to line 17 on page 3.

16. Electronic Copy Circulation	Average No. Copies Each Issue During Preceding 12 Months	No. Copies of Single Issue Published Nearest to Filing Date
a. Paid Electronic Copies	0	0
b. Total Paid Print Copies (Line 15c) + Paid Electronic Copies (Line 16a)	202	189
c. Total Print Distribution (Line 15f) + Paid Electronic Copies (Line 16a)	273	263
d. Percent Paid (Both Print & Electronic Copies) (16b divided by 16c × 100)	73.99%	71.86%

☒ I certify that 50% of all my distributed copies (electronic and print) are paid above a nominal price.

17. Publication of Statement of Ownership

☒ If the publication is a general publication, publication of this statement is required. Will be printed in the OCTOBER 2017 issue of this publication. ☐ Publication not required.

18. Signature and Title of Editor, Publisher, Business Manager or Owner: *[signature]* Stephen R. Bushing   Date 9/18/2017

STEPHEN R. BUSHING - INVENTORY DISTRIBUTION CONTROL MANAGER

I certify that all information furnished on this form is true and complete. I understand that anyone who furnishes false or misleading information on this form or who omits material or information requested on the form may be subject to criminal sanctions (including fines and imprisonment) and/or civil sanctions (including civil penalties).

PS Form **3526**, July 2014 (Page 1 of 4 (see instructions page 4)) PSN: 7530-01-000-9931   PRIVACY NOTICE: See our privacy policy on www.usps.com.

PS Form **3526**, July 2014 (Page 3 of 4)

Moving?

Make sure your subscription moves with you!

To notify us of your new address, find your **Clinics Account Number** (located on your mailing label above your name), and contact customer service at:

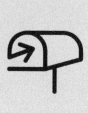

Email: journalscustomerservice-usa@elsevier.com

800-654-2452 (subscribers in the U.S. & Canada)
314-447-8871 (subscribers outside of the U.S. & Canada)

Fax number: 314-447-8029

Elsevier Health Sciences Division
Subscription Customer Service
3251 Riverport Lane
Maryland Heights, MO 63043

*To ensure uninterrupted delivery of your subscription, please notify us at least 4 weeks in advance of move.